Social Profile

Assessment of Social Participation in Children, Adolescents, and Adults

Mary V. Donohue, PhD, OT/L, FAOTA

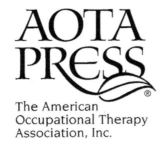

AOTA PRESS

The American
Occupational Therapy
Association, Inc.

AOTA Centennial Vision
We envision that occupational therapy is a powerful, widely recognized, science-driven, and evidence-based profession with a globally connected and diverse workforce meeting society's occupational needs.

Mission Statement
The American Occupational Therapy Association advances the quality, availability, use, and support of occupational therapy through standard-setting, advocacy, education, and research on behalf of its members and the public.

AOTA Staff
Frederick P. Somers, *Executive Director*
Christopher M. Bluhm, *Chief Operating Officer*

Chris Davis, *Director, AOTA Press*
Ashley Hofmann, *Development/Production Editor*
Victoria Davis, *Digital/Production Editor*

Beth Ledford, *Director, Marketing*
Jennifer Folden, *Marketing Specialist*
Amanda Fogle, *Marketing Specialist*

American Occupational Therapy Association, Inc.
4720 Montgomery Lane
Bethesda, MD 20814
Phone: 301–652–AOTA (2682)
TDD: 800–377–8555
Fax: 301–652–7711
www.aota.org
To order: 1–877–404–AOTA or store.aota.org

Disclaimers
This publication is designed to provided accurate and authoritative information in regard to the subject matter covered. It is sold or distributed with the understanding that the publisher is not engaged in rendering legal, accounting, or other professional service. If legal advice or other expert assistance is required, the services of a competent professional person should be sought.
—*From the Declaration of Principles jointly adopted by the American Bar Association and a Committee of Publishers and Associations*

It is the objective of the American Occupational Therapy Association to be a forum for free expression and interchange of ideas. The opinions expressed by the contributors to this work are their own and not necessarily those of the American Occupational Therapy Association.

ISBN: 978–1–56900–339–8

Library of Congress Control Number: 2012948668

Cover Design by Debra Naylor, Naylor Design, Inc., Washington, DC
Composition by Maryland Composition, Laurel, MD
Printed by Automated Graphic Systems, Inc., White Plains, MD

Contents

Items on the Flash Drive

Social Profile: Children's Version

Social Profile: Adult/Adolescent Version

Social Profile Observation Sheet for Ratings of Factors of Group Participation

About the Author

Mary V. Donohue, PhD, OT/L, FAOTA, did postdoctoral studies in assessment tool development at New York University's (NYU's) Applied Psychology Department in preparation for developing the Social Profile (SP) and carried out research for the SP in urban and suburban preschools in the New York metropolitan area. In addition, she has coordinated research using the SP in senior centers, on psychiatric units, at elementary schools, and on high school basketball courts, which involved validity, reliability, and sensitivity studies of the SP. Her research background includes using the California Psychological Inventory to study sociability, social presence, and socialization levels across several psychiatric diagnoses.

Donohue taught courses in psychosocial occupational therapy at NYU for nearly 20 years, after working with psychiatric activity groups at Hillside Hospital in Long Island, NY, for 13 years. In the day hospital and aftercare, she led occupational groups such as task skills groups, groups on psychoeducational activities of daily living and instrumental activities of daily living, women's identification groups, and furniture restoration groups.

Donohue is currently coeditor of *Occupational Therapy in Mental Health.* She also has been co-chairperson of the Metropolitan Occupational Therapy Research Committee, approving 25 Metropolitan New York District research grants for local occupational therapists. At this time, she also serves on the New York State Board for occupational therapist licensure. In 2011, she coauthored *Social Participation in Schools, Clinics and Communities* with Marilyn Cole. The SP Web site is www.Social-Profile.com. Donohue may be reached at MaryVDonohue@gmail.com.

Acknowledgments

Developing the Social Profile (SP) has been a journey in which colleagues have given input along the way. Suzanne White was so encouraging. Marie-Louise Blount shared helpful information. Peggy Swarbrick was a fellow researcher on a New York University (NYU) grant. Master occupational therapy mental health judges evaluating items included Fran Babiss, Hannah Diamond, Sharon Faust, Ellen Greer, Stanley Li, Paula McCreedy, Lori Olson, Pat Precin, Emily Chaya Weinstein, Shu-Wa Chen, Serena Wen, and Suzanne White. Helen Cohen assisted with statistical graphing. Joan Meade was my partner in assessment development in Applied Psychology class at NYU, sharing her advanced SPSS knowledge base with me for 2 semesters.

Mary Petti Weber enabled me to gain entree to carry out two research projects at Beth Israel Medical Center. Her staff, Henry Hanif and Lilya Wu Berns, gathered data using the SP in the study of its sensitivity. Ginelle John was of great assistance in embellishing the format of the SP, making disparate parts hang together. Thanks go to many NYU students who assisted in collecting data in the reliability studies. Appreciation is expressed to all the participants in the validity studies. Additionally, I would like to thank my editors at AOTA Press, Christina Davis and Ashley Hofmann, for their guidance and expertise in pulling it all together. Last, but not least, I am indebted to Malcolm Milligan for his ongoing encouragement in the writing of the SP manual.

CHAPTER 1
Overview of the Social Profile

The Social Profile (SP) is a short, descriptive psychosocial instrument designed for observational assessment of the behavioral interactions of activity groups as a whole or of individuals within an activity group. Overall, the SP measures the level of cooperation within the group or of the individual within the group. Cooperation within groups is the overarching construct of the concepts embedded in the SP.

The SP is based on the natural development of children, adolescents, and adults as they learn how to participate in social activity groups. It is used to assess whether the group or individual in the group participates appropriately at a level suitable to the activity and can shift from one level of interaction to another within a session or from day to day. It also can assess how much time those who have not developed typical interaction skills spend in developmental progression at each level. The SP also can be used to determine whether the group or individual in the group can perform at the level of social behavior appropriate for their expected developmental age level.

Multiple types of social measurement tools are currently available: general participation assessment tools (which include the SP), social network assessment tools, social role assessment tools, and social skill assessment tools. Additionally, many general assessment tools exist with subscales addressing aspects of social participation, networking, roles, and skills (Cole & Donohue, 2011). What the SP has to offer as a general participation assessment is dual measurement of an ordinal and interval nature—it is specifically designed for examining activity groups across an incremental continuum of five levels of participation and cooperation and the multiple specific social cooperative behaviors that make up these five levels. The SP provides both a general overview and a more detailed measurement of behaviors.

Children's Version

The Children's version (Appendix A) includes three levels of social interaction: (1) parallel, (2) associative, and (3) basic cooperative types of social participation in groups.

It may be used with children ages 18 months to 11 years (Mosey, 1986; Parten, 1932). This version was developed at the request of therapists, teachers, and team leaders who work with children. The Children's version of the SP is also on the flash drive included with this manual.

Adult/Adolescent Version

The Adult/Adolescent version (Appendix B), with its five levels of social interaction, may be used with persons ages 12 years or older. It includes parallel, associative, basic cooperative, supportive cooperative, and mature types of social participation in groups (Mosey, 1986; Parten, 1932).

This version can be used by therapists, teachers, and team leaders, as well as by the group members themselves, to evaluate their social participation in single sessions or across extended time periods. The Adult/Adolescent Version of the SP is also on the flash drive included with this manual.

Use of the Social Profile

The SP is intended for use by therapists, group leaders, or teachers to evaluate the interactive level of social behavioral performance in small or large groups, therapeutic groups, or groups of typically developing people.

SP scores indicate the levels at which a group or individuals perform during a session. No group is purely at one level of group interaction, even within one session, so scores are displayed across SP levels on a type of skewed or normal curve. For example, during one session, a group may carry out a sports activity, following game rules at a basic cooperative level, and then have a discussion at a supportive cooperative level focused on group and individual participatory behaviors during the game.

The SP is typically administered by a therapist, group leader, or teacher after at least a half-hour of group observation. The group or individual in the group is scored after the group has ended. At higher levels of age or function, group members can assess themselves through joint discussion and subsequently set goals accordingly.

The SP was initially designed so that therapists, clinicians, teachers, and other health professionals working in activity groups could observe and score them. Now, with items and directions presented in a more basic vocabulary and the inclusion of introductory phrases for clusters of items and lead-in questions clarifying each of the three construct pages, adolescents and adults can self-score their group.

The SP may be scored either by an individual or, preferably, through discussion, with the group jointly identifying its social participation skill levels. In any case, scorers who are members of a group are cautioned to be as objective as possible, because the purpose of self-scoring is to understand the group's current levels of participation and what the group needs to do to successfully attain new levels of participation.

Users whose vocabulary is below a sixth-grade level or who have not had experience observing and identifying elements of group work may need training. This training can be provided through lecture and discussion classes directed at classifying levels of group participation skills and by watching videos and labeling levels of behaviors. Additionally, training can be achieved through observation sessions with live groups, using rating sheets under the supervision of an experienced or trained scorer, or through use of this manual.

Scoring

A group's average score can contrast with that of an individual who is not functioning socially at the same level as most of the group. The group's average scores over multiple sessions can indicate whether it is progressing in its level of group cooperative functioning or declining in interest or interaction. The scorer can point out these average scores to the group and discuss with them how they could make an effort to change or work toward an agreed-on goal. An individual may need to move to another group whose level of current participation is closer to his or hers.

Groups or individuals in groups are assessed by means of two empirical dimensions: (1) five incremental, developmental, group, social skill levels ranging from basic to advanced group interaction on an ordinal continuum and (2) 39 Likert-scale items on which the group or individual within the group is rated, with an interval score that can be summed and distributed on a graph.

The levels and scores can be used in both clinical and empirical research. At times, the five developmental levels may be used alone for practical or clinical purposes, and the Likert-scale ratings may be used for research comparison of groups.

Continuous Rating Scale

The SP is subdivided into three sections reflecting activity group cooperation constructs: (1) activity participation, (2) social interaction, and (3) group membership and roles. Each construct is presented by asking a question:

- *Activity participation:* How do the activities influence group interaction?
- *Social interaction:* How do group members interact with each other?
- *Group membership and roles:* Do members feel they belong to the group?

Each section is divided into five levels of group participation and performance skills (Donohue, 1999; Johnson & Johnson, 2009).

Levels of Group Participation

After observing an activity group, the observer can rate the group across five levels of group participation:

1. *Parallel:* Members of the group play, move, or work side by side but do not interact with each other.
2. *Associative:* Members of the group briefly approach each other in verbal and nonverbal interactions during play, activity, or work.
3. *Basic cooperative:* Members of the group jointly select, implement, and execute longer play, activity, or work tasks for reasons of mutual self-interest in the goal, project, or fellow members.
4. *Supportive cooperative:* Members of the group are homogeneous and aim to fulfill their need for mutual emotional satisfaction, with the goals of play, activity, or work viewed as secondary. Feelings are frequently expressed.

5. *Mature:* The members of the group take turns in a variety of complementary roles to achieve the goals of the activity harmoniously and efficiently. The group combines basic cooperative and supportive cooperative interaction (Mosey, 1968, 1986; Parten, 1932).

Because this assessment tool is a profile and is used to record a range of levels of social function for a group or individual in the group, the observer needs to consider the possibility that social interactions will occur at all five levels during the observation process. Table 1.1 provides guidelines for rating group levels on the SP. These levels are calibrated so that they can be quantified and thus empirically studied.

The SP uses a Likert-type rating scale to indicate the frequency of occurrence of social behaviors across the five levels of social participation: 1 = *never,* 2 = *rarely,* 3 = *sometimes,* 4 = *frequently,* and 5 = *almost always.* In determining a rating, sometimes a decimal may be used if the rater is deliberating between two Likert scores (e.g., 2.5).

If an observer has observed a group over many sessions, he or she may mentally average the group's usual level of participation across the sessions to synthesize the group's behavioral interaction skills into one form of the SP. This synthesized perspective of the group's performance should be recorded.

Next, the average of the Likert ratings for each of the three construct areas (activity participation, social interaction, and group membership and roles) are recorded on the SP's Summary Sheet. These average scores then are transferred to the graph on the final page to create a visual profile for the group.

When reflecting on the results of this structured rating process, the observer should ask the following:

1. Did the nature of the activity influence the level of social performance?
2. Was this a typical current level or profile for the group?
3. Did the time of day, composition of the group, voluntary nature of the group, or other external social influences affect the group's profile today?

Responses to these questions may indicate the need to observe and rate the group on another day or during other activities to determine whether the group also performs at other levels (Cartwright & Zander, 1968;

Cole, 2012; Corey & Corey, 1997; Duncombe & Howe, 1995).

Summary Scores and Graph

The individual or group wanting to use the SP to rate their group's interactive participation can review the distinctions between the levels of social behaviors by using the table developed by Marilyn Cole (2012; see Table 1.1).

Creating a profile consists of observing and mentally rating and selecting Likert scores for the items on the three activity group cooperation constructs (which correspond with the topic pages of the SP): activity participation, social interaction, and group membership and roles. Next, averages of the Likert scores for each of the five levels are carried over to the Average column. If, after review, the group does not show social behaviors at all five levels, scoring just those levels that are pertinent to the particular group is acceptable and more accurate. For example, if a group scores at only the associative and the basic cooperative levels, inserting zeros for the other three areas is not necessary.

Next, the average scores for each of the five levels are transferred to each of the three corresponding columns on the Summary Sheet: activity participation, social interaction, and group membership. Again, if some levels of group social performance have not been observed in the particular group or group session, they should be omitted.

On the Summary Sheet, transferred scores should be averaged and placed in the last column, "Summary Average Topics 1, 2, 3." If meaningful to the individual scorer, he or she can calculate an average of the averages. If the score is 0 across all three topics of the parallel level, do not include it in the average summary calculation. However, if at the parallel level, one or more scores is above zero, include the average score in the average summary calculation. For example, parallel-level scores of 0, 0, and 2 across the three topics would average .67 and be included in the average summary calculation. Most often, however, the SP graph is more relevant than the summary average, because social behaviors generally occur in a range of levels. In contrast, a group of 2-year-olds may show a single level of social participation, the parallel level.

Table 1.1. Social Profile Levels and Rating Guidelines

Level	Activity Requires	Individuals Interact	Member	Leader Roles
Parallel	• Minimal sharing • Little interaction • Simple, familiar tasks	• Minimal interaction • Follow rules without disrupting group • Aware of rules	• Trusts leaders and others • Shows awareness of others	• Directive • Provides activity and support
Associative	• Engagement in short-term activities • Sharing with others • Enjoyment in interacting with others	• Seeks help with task • Willingly gives concrete assistance to others	• Shows cooperation and competition • Performance of task emphasized over relationship	• Directive • Provides choices • Encourages sharing and mutual support
Basic cooperative	• Completion of longer, more complex activities • Understanding and ownership of group goals • Basic group problem solving	• Begins to express ideas and meet others' needs • Respects rights of others and follows rules • Experiments with member roles	• Shows motivation to complete activity • Can identify and meet group goals	• Facilitative • Models need fulfillment • Takes on missing roles • Gives minimal task assistance
Supportive cooperative	• Accurately satisfying others' emotional needs • Supporting one another emotionally • Member selection of activity	• Expresses feeling • Exchanges positive and negative feelings • Shows caring for other members	• Enjoys equality and compatibility between members • Participates in mutual need satisfaction (i.e., social, emotional)	• Advisor • Connects people who are compatible • Nonauthoritative consultant
Mature	• Balance of productivity and socialization • High-level end product	• Assumes roles without prompting • Members self-lead	• Balances performance and socialization	• Coequal members • Acts as resource

Note. Courtesy of Marilyn B. Cole, MS, OTR/L, FAOTA, Professor Emerita of Occupational Therapy, Quinnipiac University. Used with permission.

Last, the averages from the Summary Sheet may be plotted on the final page of the SP, the Composite Graph, by placing points on the graph and connecting them. The scorer may plot the graph both horizontally and vertically across the five levels of social participation as well as across the three construct area columns, if this is desirable, depending on the focus of the scorer's analysis of the group (Miller, 1989; Miller, McIntire, & Lovler, 2011).

Score Interpretation

Score interpretation may look at whether the levels of social interaction were suitable for the activities and whether members could have participated at a higher level of interaction, given their backgrounds, ages, experiences, diagnoses, and lengths of treatment.

Average summary scores can be interpreted in the following way:

- 5 = *mature level of social or group participation*
- 4–5 = *supportive cooperative to mature levels of social or group participation*
- 3–4 = *basic cooperative to supportive cooperative levels of social or group participation*
- 2–3 = *associative to basic cooperative levels of social or group participation*
- 1–2 = *parallel to associative levels of social or group participation*
- 1 = *parallel level of social group participation.*

If the group leader, clinician, or researcher prefers the profile aspect of the SP, it is not necessary to average the summaries. Averaging the summaries provides a calibrated, center point regarding behaviors and performance level but may not portray the range and visualization of reporting several levels, which illustrates the range of the group's capacity for various levels of performance. Averaging the summaries is deliberately left optional to the discretion of the clinician or researcher.

Interpretation also can examine whether the follow-up group discussion focused on the levels of social interaction expected for the joint goals of the group and the individual goals of the members. Chapter 4 presents examples of group cases and interpretations of scores.

Summary

Based on the natural social development of children, adolescents, and adults, the SP serves as a descriptive psychosocial instrument designed for assessing behavioral interactions, mainly the level of cooperation. The Adult/Adolescent version examines five levels of social interaction in groups (parallel, associative, basic cooperative, supportive cooperative, and mature) for use by therapists, teachers, team leaders, and group members themselves. The Children's version includes three levels of social interaction (parallel, associative, and basic cooperative). In both versions, social participation can be assessed in a single session or across extended time periods.

CHAPTER 2   Theoretical Basis of the Social Profile

The basis for the Social Profile (SP) is the psychosocial context of the human personality developing sociability, social presence, and socialization (Gough, 1987). This chapter examines the origins of Social Participation Theory, Parten's (1932) ideas regarding social participation, related models of social learning, and the assumptions of the SP.

Origins of Social Participation

The theoretical base underlying the SP is the major construct of social participation. In 1932, Mildred Parten laid out a conceptual continuum of the development of social participation. This continuum was defined by six classifications, or concepts of play, consisting of interactive activities in a group, which she organized into two categories:

Preparatory participation:
1. Unoccupied
2. Onlooker
3. Solitary.

Levels of interaction:
4. Parallel
5. Associative
6. Cooperative.

Preparatory participation behaviors occurring near or in a group of preschool children include a child's remaining idle at the perimeter of the group, watching others in the group, or ignoring the group while playing alone. A child playing close to other children in a group while still playing independently is engaged in *parallel play. Associative play* involves behaviors such as sharing materials and equipment in brief encounters. Children may momentarily engage with other children in similar or the same activities. During associative play, children may follow each other around in unorganized activities. The concept of *cooperative play* consists of organized activity in which

children follow the norms of a game, take turns, role play, complete a task, and support other children's activities (Parten, 1932).

According to Parten (1932), in the sequential development of social participation, the three purposeful concepts of parallel, associative, and cooperative behaviors are age-related. As Parten also indicated, these parallel, associative, and cooperative behaviors overlap as people practice levels of interaction, and they are not abandoned as a child develops but rather are manifested again in various situations as appropriate.

Parten's (1932) empirical data showed that the construct of social participation consists of a spectrum of behavioral classifications, as depicted in Figure 2.1, which shows the six concepts of play dimensions. Her work also provided principles for future confirmation of the relationship of age to social development and the overlapping nature of social stages in development of participation skills, which are reflected in the SP's formatting as a graded, graphic profile.

Geselle (1940) amplified Parten's principles of social participation development, explaining in great detail the chronological trends found in multiple individuals as they matured. Later, Gough (1987) developed the California Psychological Inventory, which has three subscales devoted to social participation in later childhood, adolescence, and adulthood: (1) sociability, (2) social presence, and (3) socialization. These subscales reflect a progression in social behaviors that gradually demands a more mature involvement in society.

Sociability is the capacity and desire to enjoy the company of others with informal affability and outgoing friendliness. *Social presence,* in its positive mode, is the capacity to interact with others with poise, spontaneity, and self-confidence. *Socialization* refers to a person's development of social maturity, stability, and rectitude and manifestation of honesty, industriousness, and responsibility in his or her life roles. Gough's (1987) concepts of social participation to some

Figure 2.1. Social participation and age.

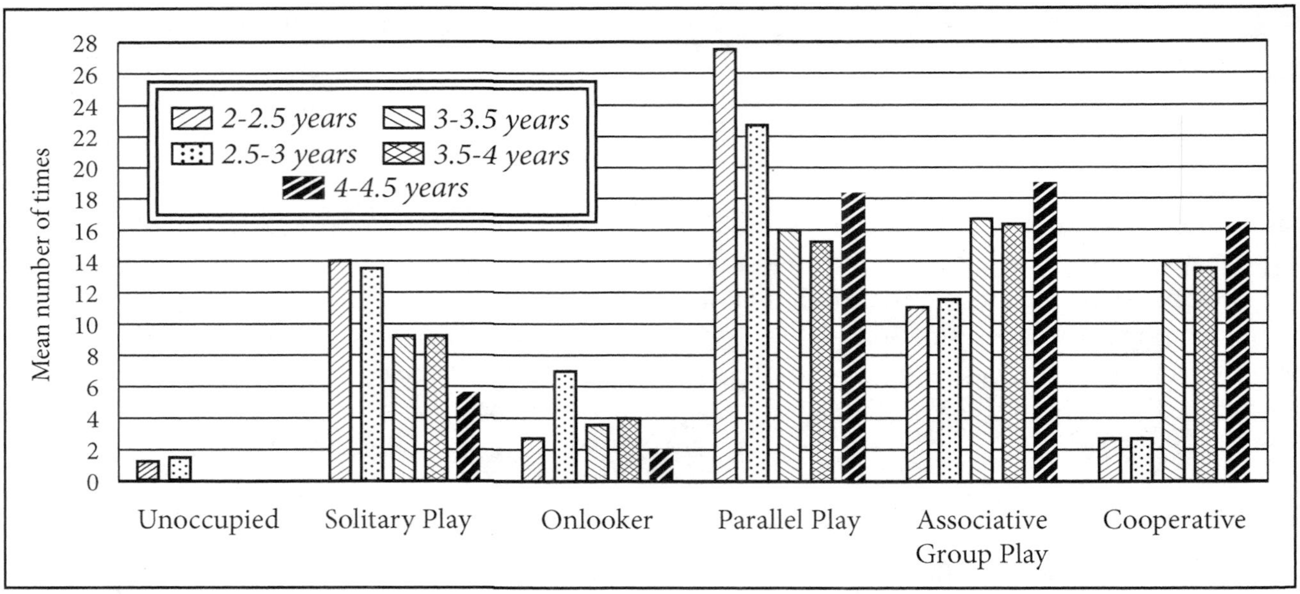

Note. From "Social Participation Among Pre-School Children," by M. B. Parten, 1932, *Journal of Abnormal and Social Psychology, 27,* p. 260. Copyright © 1932, by the American Psychological Association. Used with permission.

extent parallel the SP's basic cooperative, supportive cooperative, and mature levels of social behavior.

Mosey (1968) undertook the direct expansion of Parten's (1932) theoretical construct of social participation in her article "Recapitulation of Ontogenesis," and she further refined Parten's theoretical frame of reference (Mosey, 1986). Mosey extended the continuum of Parten's three social participation levels by adding two more levels, supportive cooperative and mature.

Although Mosey (1986) referred to *social interaction* rather than to *social participation,* she built on Parten's (1932) parallel, associative, and cooperative levels of social behavior. Mosey retained Parten's parallel level; the associative level became the *project level* to indicate that brief group projects are engaged in during associative play behaviors. This choice put the emphasis on participation in the activity rather than on social participation. The SP uses *association* because observations of preschool groups have revealed that association is the natural emergence of brief social interactions among preschool children who are moving from the partial isolation of parallel play to a more advanced level of social participation (see discussion of participation levels in Chapter 1; Donohue, 2003, 2005, 2006).

Mosey (1968, 1986) also chose to divide Parten's (1932) cooperative level into two parts, (1) egocentric cooperative and (2) cooperative, believing that the development step from the associative level to the cooperative level was too sudden. *Egocentric cooperative* implies that this type of cooperation is self-serving. Much of childhood involves consolidating gains in social participation, such as experimenting with group activities, assuming a role as a group member, and organizing games and activities (Donohue, 2003, 2005, 2006). Reflecting a more positive expansion of social participation behaviors throughout childhood, the egocentric cooperative concept is labeled *basic cooperative* in the SP (Donohue, 2003, 2005, 2006).

Mosey (1968, 1986) labeled adolescents' social participation as *cooperative group-level interaction,* which is an apt description of adolescents' interaction. Often distinguished by homogeneous membership and emotional expression of needs, mutual camaraderie, and recognition of feelings, the cooperative group-level interaction task sometimes takes second place to social interaction. The SP labels this level of social participation as *supportive cooperative,* which conveys an advanced ability to recognize individuals' personal contribution to the group (Donohue, 2010b). Lifton (1966) described mature behaviors as self-directed, patient, expressing emotions in socially acceptable ways, and sensitive to the feelings of others.

Exhibit 2.1. Definitions of Social Profile Concepts

Parallel participation: The members of the group play, move, or work side by side but do not interact with each other.

Associative participation: The members of the group approach each other briefly in verbal and nonverbal interactions during play, activity, or work.

Basic cooperative participation: The members of the group jointly select, implement, and execute longer play, activity, or work tasks for reasons of mutual self-interest in the goal, project, or fellow members.

Supportive cooperative participation: The members of the group are homogeneous and aim to fulfill their need for mutual emotional satisfaction; the goals of play, activity, or work are viewed as secondary. Feelings are frequently expressed.

Mature participation: The members of the group are heterogeneous, taking turns in a variety of complementary roles to achieve the goals of the activity harmoniously and efficiently. The group combines basic cooperative and supportive cooperative interaction.

This concept of an adult level of social participation also incorporated a goal-oriented element, so Mosey (1968, 1986) labeled this concept *mature*. In the SP, the mature level incorporates aspects of both the basic and the supportive cooperative levels. Definitions of SP concepts are presented in Exhibit 2.1.

An interesting study of social participation was published. In *The Social Animal*, Brooks (2011) popularized interest in and intently studied social participation, using a descriptive, lifelong case study type of presentation to look at loving interactions. In 2010, Mezrich detailed the founding of Facebook, a social network, which expanded the focus of interaction to the Internet, with some paradoxical results in the definitions of *social* and *group*. In *Connected*, Christiakis and Fowler (2011) contribute to the discussion of groups and the influence of friends with diagrammatic analysis using sociograms. Their analysis of network friends online questions how many of them are close friends.

The Social Cure (Jetten, Haslam, & Haslam, 2012) presented an international perspective on the identity, health, and general well-being of people who join social networks. Authors from Canada, England, Australia, Spain, Scotland, and Germany were included, indicat-ing the value of social contacts in international settings. Social outreach and organization carried out by the women of Liberia showed how sisterhood, prayer, and sex changed their nation at war. One of the leaders, Leymah Gbowee, told her story in *Mighty Be Our Powers* (Gbowee & Mithers, 2011). She and two of her colleagues received a Nobel Peace Prize in 2011 for their joint work and leadership achieved against all odds.

Continuous Use of the Concept

Mosey's (1986) concept of social interaction contin-ues to be used in psychosocial occupational therapy group process books (Bruce & Borg, 2002; Cole, 2012; Posthuma, 2002; Schwartzberg, Howe, & Barnes, 2008). Her ideas regarding change are presented as guidelines for practice, indicating that the five levels of participation behaviors may be achieved by practicing goals and behaviors in activity groups led according to the guidelines for leaders presented in Table 2.1.

Mosey's (1986) group interaction skill develop-ment also included the principle of using groups as an opportunity to model social behaviors at the five con-cept levels, with group members modeling appropriate behaviors for each other. Another principle was to in-corporate a discussion of behavioral goals at the end of activity group meetings to consolidate gains or move members along in the social participation progression.

In the 1980s, many investigators became interested in the emergence of associative and cooperative behav-iors in children attending preschool in comparison with that of children who did not. Field (1984), Guralnick and Groom (1987, 1988), and Howes (1988) observed that children who attended preschool were able to engage in associative and cooperative behaviors with other chil-dren to a greater extent than children who did not. In 1981, Hertz-Lazarowitz, Feitelson, Zahavi, and Hartup used Parten's (1932) six categories of social participa-tion, noting that kindergarten students participated in significantly smaller groups than first-grade students. Krantz (1982) examined sociometric awareness of per-ceived popularity among preschool children by exam-ining their communicative ability using Parten's (1932) social participation continuum.

By way of contrast, in 1993, Saracho researched Parten's (1932) concepts using factor analysis in a

Table 2.1. Adaptation of Mosey's Group Levels

Group Level	Developmental Group Issues	Roles and Behaviors	Activities and Environment	Leader's Role
Parallel (ages 18 months–2 years)	• Initial levels of basic trust; tolerates play in presence of others	• Level just above an aggregate of people • Some minimal mutual stimulation and awareness • Not disruptive • Group membership roles • Minimal verbal and nonverbal exchange	• Minimal sharing of tasks • Sufficient materials for all • Familiar activities encourage interaction	• Selects activity to meet safety, love, and esteem needs • Reinforces parallel skills • Provides task assistance
Associative (ages 2–4 years)	• Beginning shared interaction: some cooperation and competition • Task is paramount	• Seek some task assistance from others • Give concrete assistance willingly • Understand give-and-take in helping roles	• Engage in short-term tasks • Can join in sharable tasks • Promotes enjoyment of task	• Activity selected reinforces desired behaviors • Encourages subgroupings • Helps group select tasks • Encourages trial and error • Fosters cooperation and competition
Basic cooperative (ages 5–7 years)	• Joint task interaction with self-interest manifested • Identify and meet group norms and goals	• Enjoy meeting some needs of self or group at a basic level • Experiment with group member roles • Perceive group membership as a right; respect for others' rights given	• Select longer, more complex tasks • Activities reflect norms and goals • Activities can be completed • Foster group problem solving	• Role model love and safety need fulfillment • Give minimal assistance • Serve as resource person • Take on missing roles
Supportive cooperative (ages 9–12 years)	• Enjoy as homogeneous, compatible membership and camaraderie • Participate in mutual need satisfaction	• Encourage self-expression • Express positive and negative feelings • Recognize and fulfill safety, love, and belonging needs of others	• Satisfy others' needs accurately • Task is secondary to need fulfillment • Express activities selected	• Share responsibility for reinforcing behavior • Connect people who are compatible • Nonauthoritative consultant
Mature (ages 15–18 years)	• Maintain balance between task and maintenance behaviors	• Assess and assume roles as needed • Heterogeneous roles	• Balance between emotional and task needs • Near-perfect end product	• Shared leadership: Therapist is peer

Note. Adapted by Donohue with White, Blount, and Swarbrick from *Psychosocial Components of Occupational Therapy* by A. C. Mosey, 1986, New York: Raven Press. From "Theoretical Bases of Mosey's Group Interaction Skills," by M. V. Donohue, 1999, *Occupational Therapy International*, Vol. 6, p. 41. Copyright © 1999, by Whurr Publishers. Used with permission.

study of 2,400 preschool children and found that parallel (84% of variance) and associative behaviors (16% of variance) were most prevalent. The factor analysis did not detect cooperative behaviors. Saracho's challenge to Parten's work has not been replicated.

To further confirm Parten's (1932) ideas, in 1994 Henninger examined outdoor play among children, evaluating social and cognitive aspects. He observed that all levels of play—parallel, associative, and cooperative—were found when studying the behaviors of children. In the same year, Garnier and Latour (1994) researched the continuum of parallel, associative, and cooperative behaviors. They found that cooperative behaviors emerged earlier than the expected age of 3 to 3.5 years (Parten, 1932), with a gradual increase in frequency, depth, and complexity as the years pass. More cooperative behaviors were associated with a younger age group than in most other studies ($p = .0021$).

Looking at the social and cognitive behaviors of children in day care centers, Petrakos and Howe (1996) focused on solitary play during free-play periods to evaluate the role of environmental design in encouraging participation. They found that more group interaction took place in centers designed for groups (57.3%) than centers designed for solitary or parallel activity (42.7%). In the same year, Fantuzzo and colleagues (1996) studied children in Head Start programs to assess a peer treatment program for children who had been physically abused or neglected. They were able to use Parten's (1932) three levels to distinguish between children who had or had not been abused or neglected, because the children who had been abused or neglected more often were involved in solitary play ($F[1, 44] = 6.13$, $p < .05$). Children in positive relationships were more involved in participatory play than children who were exposed to physical abuse and neglect ($F[1, 44] = 12.96$, $p < .001$).

Focusing on one of Parten's (1932) principles regarding the multiple levels of social participation acquired in sequence by preschool-age children, Robinson, Anderson, Porter, Hart, and Wouden-Miller (2003) examined sequential transition patterns among parallel–aware and cooperative–social states of play. They found bidirectionality of movement among behavioral levels of play in preschool children after the children had advanced in overall performance from onlooker to parallel to cooperative behavioral levels in earlier development, indicating that some children return to earlier, comfortable levels of social participation.

Summarizing Parten's (1932) work more recently, Hughes (2009) and Santrock (2007) emphasized the developmental aspects of children's play patterns. Santrock used a topical approach to lifespan aspects of Parten's classic study of play, and Hughes focused on the relationship of play to children's physical, social, intellectual, and emotional growth. Their presentations of Parten's theory were based on the findings of most researchers whose work confirmed Parten's study, indicating a continuous progression in social skill development.

Social Learning Models

In 1940, psychologists Neal Miller and John Dollard wrote about social learning, which is achieved through imitation of other humans' behavior. Psychologist Albert Bandura (1977) theorized about social learning, arguing that "learning would be exceedingly laborious, not to mention hazardous, if people had to rely solely on the effects of their own action to inform them what to do. Fortunately, most human behavior is learned observationally through modeling" (p. 22). He then added the aspect of cognition to modeling when he pointed out that modeling is not just a matter of mimicry but is more a process of abstracting rules (Bandura, 1986). Bandura (1973) also studied the social learning aspects of aggression and stimulated an ongoing debate about movies' and television's influence on violent behavior.

Related to Bandura's (1977) Social Learning Theory, psychologist Lev Vygotsky's Social Development Theory suggests that people learn by imitating others' behaviors. Vygotsky's (1978) principle of *social interaction* states that

> every function in the child's cultural development appears twice: first, on the social level and later, on the individual level; first between people *(interpsychological)* and then inside the child *(intrapsychological)*. . . . All the higher functions originate as actual relationships between individuals. (p. 57, *italics added*)

Likewise, Jean Lave's (1988) situated learning is a derivative of Bandura's Social Learning Theory and emphasizes context and culture. Drawing on her background as a social anthropologist, Lave viewed learners as immersed in a community of behaviors through collaborative social interaction and social organization of knowledge.

Rao, Moely, and Lockman (1987) showed preschool children a social-modeling film depicting appropriate social behavior and found that the social participation scores of preschool children who were usually withdrawn increased in contrast to those of children shown a film about animals. The films were shown on two occasions to each group in an effort to improve social participation through a planned social-modeling intervention.

International Classification of Functioning, Disability and Health

In 2001, the World Health Organization (WHO) addressed the concepts of activities and social participation in the *International Classification of Functioning, Disability and Health (ICF)*. Chapter 7, "Interpersonal Interactions and Relationships," described a range of relationships from strangers; to formal and structured business, political, and religious relationships; and to family, relatives, lovers, and friends as being part of a healthy life, in a contextually and socially appropriate manner. Specifically, people were encouraged to show consideration and esteem when responding to others' feelings. Chapter 9, "Community, Social and Civic Life," described healthy people as engaging in organized social life outside the family, such as involvement in charitable organizations, clubs, or professional social organizations incorporating recreation, leisure, religion, spirituality, human rights, political life, and citizenship.

In 2007, WHO developed the *International Classification of Functioning, Disability and Health for Children and Youth (ICF–CY)*, which includes Parten's (1932) levels of participatory functioning. Spanning these two versions of the *ICF*, the SP encourages and measures social participation in health for adults and in school for children.

Social–Emotional Learning

Schools have many programs designed to foster *social–emotional learning (SEL)*, or the process of identifying emotions in oneself and in others to build positive re-lationships for interactions at school, home, and work and with friends.

Schools establish SEL programs to promote the construct of positive social participation. Incorporated in the SEL construct are the concepts of healthy environments, recognizing and self-regulating emotions, problem solving in interpersonal situations, and fostering social relationships. Children and adults are encouraged to learn skills to calm themselves when they are overwhelmed with emotion; to approach others in a caring manner; and to build positive relationships at school, at home, and in the community.

The Illinois State Board of Education (2008) developed SEL standards for the Illinois Learning Standards, including principles and goals such as the following:

- Develop self-awareness and self-management skills to achieve school and life success;
- Use social awareness and interpersonal skills to establish and maintain positive relationships; and
- Demonstrate decision making and responsible behaviors in personal, school, and community contexts.

Two centers founded to promote social–emotional competence are the Collaborative for Academic, Social, and Emotional Learning in Chicago (www.casel.org) and the National School Climate Center in New York (www.schoolclimate.org). The National School Climate Center's purpose is to create a climate for learning participation in democracy and in development of well-being; it promotes working together to improve a school's climate and culture as a place in which the total school community can share and acquire knowledge from one another by working collaboratively, which can be achieved by being aware of the needs of all members of the school community (Cohen, 2006; Devine, Cohen, & Elias, 2007).

Zins and Elias (2007) described children's needs, and Cohen (2004) discussed the concept of caring classrooms, which expands on SEL and how to establish an appropriate learning environment. Additionally, the American Educational Research Association (www.aera.net) has created a special interest group on SEL.

Social Capital

Social capital refers to connections within and between social networks in business, economics, organizational behavior, political science, public health, sociology, and environmental management (Portes, 1998). At a practical level, Hanifan (1916) stated that social capital consists of aspects of people's daily life, such as cooperation, camaraderie, understanding, and social interaction among family, friends, and neighbors.

The construct of social capital continues to expand through international dissemination (Centers for Disease Control and Prevention, 2008; Coleman, 1988; Fukuyama, 1995, 1999; World Bank, 2008). Social capital makes up the fabric of the larger community social profile.

Assumptions of the Social Profile

Parten's (1932) and Mosey's (1968, 1986) models are based on developmental theory and assume that human growth skills advance with increasing age (see Figure 2.1 and Table 2.1). Freud (Brown, 1971) and Erikson (1968) both assumed that developmental stages could not be skipped if psychosexual or psychosocial development was to unfold. Another assumption of developmental models is that plateaus or crises (Erikson, 1968) sometimes occur that apparently stall progress but are occasionally needed for gestation and gathering of strength before a new developmental growth spurt can occur.

Developmental theory accepts the premise that individuals may advance farther in some areas of human skill than in others, and developmental constructs allow for individual progress through specialization of skills (Piaget, 1956), so that other skill areas are left undeveloped or underdeveloped. It is a rare individual who can simultaneously expand multiple areas of human skill to achieve a level of expertise across the board (Schwartzberg, 2002).

These assumptions apply to the interpretation of the SP (Precin, 1999). The SP's developmental levels include plateaus, and a person does not spend an equal amount of time at each level of social ability over the years (Table 2.1). Even at the theoretical level, people should expect continuous but variable progress in advancing skills and detect this progress through general observation (Schwartzberg, Howe, & McDermott, 1982). People at each social participation skill level need exposure, practice, and saturation before moving on to the next

social–behavioral stage. A change in the environment that demands a developmental adaptation or activity might propel an individual forward to the next stage.

Assessment Incorporating Assumptions Observed During Research

Some assumptions about social participation that have surfaced through research need to be empirically tested (Neufeld, 2004). One assumption is that the activity can shape the environment and elicit participation behaviors at a given level. Formal studies aside (Donohue, 2003, 2005, 2006; see Chapter 3), clinical and educational observations are described in Exhibit 2.2.

As Exhibit 2.2 shows, the degree of interaction gradually increases over the first three levels of activity. It then expands to insightful recognition and understanding of feelings and ethical norms in oneself and in others at the supportive cooperative and mature levels. In addition, certain activities promote, induce, or elicit given levels of social participation if the individual in the group is ready to perform social skills at that level. In designing activity groups, the therapist should keep this assumption in mind (O'Neil & Perez, 2007; Remocker & Sherwood, 1999).

Although Parten's (1932) model indicates a gradual introduction to various social skill levels of participation while earlier skill levels are sustained, Mosey's (1968, 1986) model appears to imply that the skill levels exist only at certain age ranges. One assumption coming out of SP studies (Donohue, 2003, 2005, 2006) is that the levels of social participation are not mutually exclusive (Passi, 1998). Once an individual is able to socially interact at a particular level, his or her performance in a given session can manifest at several of the levels. Thus, the SP is designed to measure the continuum of social participation skills across a spectrum of activities. Groups and individuals are anticipated to manifest several levels of social participation performance, meaning that, for example, during one session a group may function at the parallel level 25% of the time, at the associative level 25% of the time, and at the basic cooperative level 50% of the time. A graph of the group's profile would therefore display these multiple levels of performance of social participation for that period of time (Jackson & Arbesman, 2005; Kim, Kim, & Kaslak, 2005; see Appendixes A and B).

Exhibit 2.2. Typical Activities Observed in Social Profile Levels of Group Participation

Parallel
- Children use toys, scooters, phones, and bikes separately without interaction.
- Children play next to each other in a sand box, pouring sand into cups.
- Adults work at separate computer stations or exercise in lines on mats following a leader at the front of the class without interacting.
- Seniors listen to a lecture on prevention of illness.

Associative
- Children briefly build a tower together using building blocks.
- Children put chairs in a line and get on the "bus" for a brief ride.
- Children briefly talk on phones.
- Two girls push a stroller together.
- Adults engage in a pass-the-ball game in a circle, calling the names of those to whom they throw the ball.
- Teens have brief smart phone contact.
- Adult patients play the parachute game, calling out each other's names as they exchange seats under the parachute.
- Adult commuters waiting for a train briefly talk about the weather.
- Office workers joke at the coffee or copy machine.

Basic Cooperative
- Children say, "Let's dress up together and play make believe," "Let's build a fort out of these cartons," or "Let's have a tea party."
- Adult patients in a cooking group each prepare a different vegetable for a salad, with a little conversation while working.
- Many politicians work at this level: "What can you do for me? What can I do for you?"
- An inpatient group plans a holiday party or weekend activity.

Supportive Cooperative
- Teens make decorations for a dance or express feelings about the lyrics of a song.
- Informal adolescent cliques hang out in groups without adults.
- Adults describe feelings about characters in a book during a book club meeting.
- Seniors discuss feelings about ailments and prescription prices.
- People participate in Alcoholics Anonymous, Narcotics Anonymous, Gamblers Anonymous, and other 12-step support groups.

Mature
- Parents of children with learning disabilities coach each other in a multifamily support group; parents participate in parent–teacher associations.
- Adult patients in a community group meeting discuss forming a group after discharge to help them stay clean of substances.
- Friends plan a weekend vacation.

Another assumption of the SP is that adults may function at the parallel level of social participation when their circumstances and activities warrant parallel interaction. For example, in an office pool of computer cubicles, the work performed is in parallel mode in relationship to other office workers in neighboring cubicles. During this activity and in this setting would not be the time for adults to use their social skills to hang out by the copier, exchanging feelings appropriate for a supportive cooperative group, unless the conversation is a brief exchange. An organized office party would be the time for a supportive cooperative and mature group interaction.

Summary

The SP can be used to assess the levels of participation in SEL (Cole & Donohue, 2011) of groups in classrooms, extracurricular activities, afterschool programs, class meetings, and assemblies. The SP also may be used to assess social interaction levels in the community in churches, synagogues, temples, sports, clubs, professional groups, and legislative bodies. SEL methods may then be used to work on developing social group goals revealed in the assessment process, as delineated earlier in this chapter.

CHAPTER 3 Development of the Social Profile

The evaluation of social participation has been based on observation of familial, educational, clinical, and community interactional behaviors, as well as on review of concepts of social behavior in the literature (Cole & Donohue, 2011; Donohue, 2010a). Working from these sources, a heuristically appropriate assessment tool was created by means of item construction and validation, determining the Social Profile's (SP) reliability and sensitivity.

Item Construction

Item construction involves reviewing relevant written sources and searching the universe of significant terms by observing and interviewing people familiar with the topic under study to select valid statements designed to analyze and summarize the topic's core. Developing items for the SP began with a two-pronged approach: (1) concepts from the work of Parten (1932) and Mosey (1968) and (2) observations of groups of all ages engaged in a variety of activities. Parten's and Mosey's work is discussed in Chapter 2.

Preschool groups of specific ages and various cultural and socioeconomic backgrounds were formally observed in 36 group sessions in 8 metropolitan and suburban settings. These children, who were developing typically, were observed during free-play activities they selected, with the aim of illustrating participation behaviors that were natural or typical for these children's stage of social interaction. The author and fellow researchers were looking for behaviors that fit the schema of Parten (1932) and Mosey (1968): parallel play, associative or project play, and basic cooperative play.

Elementary and middle school children from a range of socioeconomic and cultural backgrounds were observed engaging in self-chosen activities on playgrounds and in gymnasiums, lunchrooms, and classroom art groups in nine rural, suburban, and city settings in four geographic areas of metropolitan New York and New Jersey. The author examined typical social participation and looked for nontypical social interaction behaviors.

Groups of typically developing junior high and high school students also were observed during self-selected activities on sports fields and in gyms, lunchrooms, and club groups in six settings in four types of rural, suburban, and city neighborhoods. The adolescent groups were examined for socially acceptable and atypical behaviors using the full version of the SP, because clinically and theoretically adolescents are expected to have achieved the supportive cooperative level of interaction, which is on the Adult/Adolescent version of the SP but not on the Children's version (Donohue, 2003, 2005, 2006; Mosey, 1986).

Subscales

The theoretical constructs of Parten (1932) and Mosey (1968, 1986) were organized into three areas: (1) activity participation, (2) social interaction, and (3) group membership and roles. The Activity Participation subscale is placed first in the SP because it incorporates the most concrete construct and concepts and its concepts are the easiest to observe. The Social Interaction subscale was placed next in sequence because observers can see participation behaviors quite readily. The Group Membership and Roles subscale is last because it includes the most abstract concepts and items (Donohue, 2003, 2005, 2006).

Sensitivity of Items for Observation of Social Participation Behaviors

Thirty-nine items were developed from Mosey's (1986) group levels (discussed in Chapter 2) and the previously mentioned observations. The items were first field tested in five preschools in outer urban and suburban classrooms with children ages 2 to 6 years in free-play activities and compiled using the first three levels of the SP. The apparent ease of identifying social participation behaviors with the SP merited statistical examination of the first three levels of social participation. (This study is described later in this chapter in the sections on "Analysis of Internal Consistency Reliability of Items" and "Content

Validity.") Subsequently, graduate occupational therapy students and psychosocial occupational therapists also used the SP in preschools, senior community groups, a religious community dance group of middle-age women, and reliability studies at psychiatric hospitals.

Groups with sufficient maturity and insight may want to use the SP to study their own groups (Jackson, Carlson, Mandel, Zemke, & Clark, 1998), for example, adolescent sports teams, middle-age adult recreational groups, and senior community groups. The feedback provided by the observers and self-scorers in senior community groups indicated that the SP's length was manageable for rating their groups accurately without tiring. They found that the Likert scale provided enough of a range to rate each social behavioral item with ease (Donohue, 2001).

However, adult self-scorers in two groups initially found some of the vocabulary in the early items to be unfamiliar. Their feedback was incorporated by changing the wording of items to more familiar phrases and by introducing each cluster or level of items with an overview statement in bold. Several students and adult self-scorers suggested introducing each construct page of items with a question, in addition to the title, to provide an overview of what the observer or self-scorer needed to focus on for that page. Incorporating these suggestions further clarified the SP.

Analysis of Items' Internal Consistency Reliability

In the first study, 21 preschool groups of typically developing children were examined using the first three levels of the SP: parallel participation, associative participation, and basic cooperative participation (Donohue, 2003). An analysis of internal consistency was used to compare each SP item with every other item to judge the items' reliability and determine whether they had sufficient cohesion.

Using an alpha coefficient item analysis, the SP's internal consistency reliability was examined using item–total statistics. A moderate level of internal reliability, .7073, was found by determining the overall alpha reliability coefficient. In an item analysis, a moderate level of internal reliability is desirable; a high alpha coefficient would indicate that some items need to be discarded because they are too similar (Spector, 1992). Applying a Bonferroni correction for the alpha coefficient resulted in a more accurate and highly significant coefficient: $\alpha = .05/4 = \alpha = .0125$, $p < .000$.

To determine whether any SP items needed to be removed because their content was too similar, two experimental item analyses were carried out. The item analysis outcomes did not indicate a need to remove an item; the deletion of any item would have resulted in only a slightly higher alpha coefficient. That the coefficients for item reliability were closely related, but not identical, indicated that the SP provides a univariate measure of social participation capable of reliably measuring the concepts it claims to measure. The item reliability result reinforces that the SP is appropriate for evaluating the participation of members of a social group. The sample size, 21 groups, is considered an adequate number of groups for measuring a scale's internal reliability (Donohue, 2003).

Validity: Content, Construct, and Criterion

Three types of validity tests were used to analyze the accuracy and meaningfulness of the items of the SP as relevant to the concepts of social participation in groups: (1) content, (2) construct, and (3) criterion validity. Factor and cluster analysis is also discussed.

Content validity

In the same study previously described (Donohue, 2003), 11 expert judges who were experienced psychosocial activity group leaders examined the SP's content validity. These judges evaluated the clarity, appropriateness, and sequence of and need for items included in the SP. These judges were also familiar with the concepts of Parten (1932) and Mosey (1968, 1986) embedded in a developmental frame of reference of group participation and interaction skills in activity groups (see Chapter 2, Table 2.1).

At this point in time, the SP was much longer, composed of as many items as possible to incorporate the universe of concepts relevant to the levels of social participation. In their evaluation, the judges labeled items as *essential, useful but not essential,* or *not essential.* They rated many items as essential and useful but perceived the SP to be too long. By selecting the most relevant conceptual items, the judges greatly reduced the SP's length so that the items most important to each level of social participation could be sequentially rank ordered within each cluster and subscale (Bernard, 2000; Carmines & Zeller, 1991; Cohen, Swerdlik, & Phillips, 1995; Deci & Ryan, 2000).

A validity study of Parten's (1932) and Mosey's (1968) concepts was undertaken to develop the schema found in Table 2.1, the four-scale adaptation of Mosey's (1986) group developmental levels. This process was also a part of the examination of the SP's content validity, analyzing how the five social-level concepts related to the constructs of activity environment or participation, developmental group issues, social interaction and role behaviors, and group membership.

It should be pointed out that as content validity was scrutinized, the labels for the five levels were also examined. Some of the labels were changed for the sake of clarity and impartiality. Parten (1932) called the second level of social participation *associative,* describing how children begin to associate as they move from the parallel play stage to attempting interaction with others. Although Mosey (1986) called this the *project* level, occupational therapists who currently use this model have found *associative* to be more self-explanatory of what happens in this exploratory stage of social development.

Mosey (1968) took Parten's (1932) third level of participation, cooperative, and divided it into two levels: a third level, *egocentric cooperative,* and a fourth level, *cooperative.* However, in circumstances in which a group wants to use the SP to discuss and evaluate its usual level of participation, consideration was given to the idea that no one would want to label himself or herself as egocentric cooperative. As a result, the third level was labeled *basic cooperative* and the fourth, *supportive cooperative.* The fundamental difference between the two types of cooperation is that Level 3 operates on the basis of mutually beneficial interaction, usually following rules of the organization, game, or setting.

Through the judges' review, the SP was reduced from 252 items to 166 items. The judges maintained that the five group-level concepts of the SP followed a meaningful interactive progression of group social skills development. Because clinicians critiqued the 166-item version as still being too long, repetitious and nonessential items were removed before progressing to further validity studies.

Construct validity

Age groups were used as one construct against which to measure developmental skills in activity group

participation. First, in a study (Donohue, 2003) of 21 groups, 242 typically developing preschool children engaged in free play, and the validity of the sequence of levels of group interactive ability was examined as the children grew older. Parallel behaviors occurred most frequently in 2- to 3-year-olds ($M = 3.2$), associative behaviors were found most often in 4- to 5-year olds ($M = 3.43$), and basic cooperative behaviors were observed more often in 5-year-olds ($M = 2.72$). These trends are shown in the mean Likert ratings displayed in Table 3.1. Although 5-year-olds exhibited basic cooperative behaviors more often than other age groups, they continued to demonstrate a higher level of associative behaviors ($M = 3.31$) than of basic cooperative behaviors (Bernard, 2012), thus illustrating that 5-year-olds are most likely still transitioning, frequently using both the associative and basic cooperative participatory levels of group performance skills (Bredenkamp & Copple, 2009).

This result and Figure 3.1 demonstrate the need for a profile to measure how children move through the levels of participatory behavior, consolidating skills in a lower level while simultaneously experimenting with skills in a higher level (Burns & Grove, 2009). Figure 3.1 shows that parallel participation behaviors decline in frequency among 2- to 4-year-olds. Associative behaviors increased among 2- to 4-year-olds, declining only slightly in 5-year-olds. Basic cooperative behaviors were initiated at age 3, becoming stronger at ages 4 and 5 (Donohue, 2003).

Table 3.1. Mean Likert Ratings and Analysis of Variance for Four Age Groups and Across Three Group Interaction Behaviors

Age Group	Parallel	Associative	Basic Cooperative
2	3.2	0.58	0.00
3	2.36	2.38	0.55
4	0.75	3.43	1.98
5	0.20	3.31	2.72
F	22.675	8.063	9.99
p	.000	.001	.000

Note. N = 21 groups (242 children).

Figure 3.1. Four age groups across three levels of social behavior.

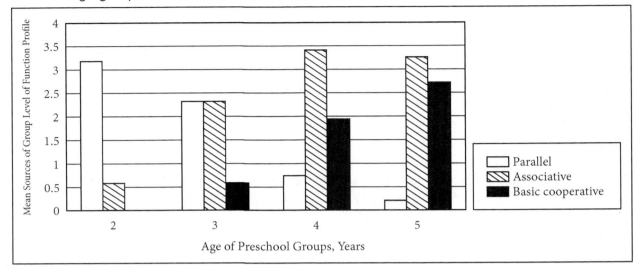

Note. N = 21 groups (242 children).

For the sake of confirming these differences among the three group-level abilities displayed by preschool children, an analysis of variance (ANOVA) was performed for the 21 groups (242 children) using the SP. In a between-group analysis of the four age groups (2-, 3-, 4, and 5-year-olds), the ANOVA interactions were significant, as can be seen in Table 3.1 (parallel level, p = .000; associative level, p = .001; basic cooperative level, p = .000; Carmines & Zeller, 1991).

An item at the parallel level on the original SP asked whether every child had sufficient materials. Another 4 × 27 × 3 (Age Group × Item × Level) ANOVA of the four ages across the 27 items for the 3 levels indicated that this item had low significance (.082) in contrast to other expected significance levels. The presence or absence of materials is not under the children's control, so this item was removed from the SP, resulting in 39 items (Nachmias & Nachmias, 2008).

This study's (Donohue, 2003) results also were examined using a Spearman rank order correlation to research the relationship between the known age groups and expected rank order of behavioral group levels in activity groups of preschool children (see Table 3.2). With 12 groups (n = 131 children) ages 2 to 3 years, 10 groups (n = 134 children) ages 3 to 4 years, and 9 groups (n = 111 children) ages 4 to 5 years, this analysis sought to highlight the correlation of these age

groups with the parallel, associative, and basic cooperative levels of participation behaviors, respectively. Age ranges were used because social participation is projected to develop gradually.

The correlation between 2- and 3-year-olds and parallel-level behaviors was r =.8805, p = .0000; between 3- and 4-year-olds and associative-level behaviors, r =.7139, p = .0003; and between 4- and 5-years-olds and basic cooperative–level behaviors, r =.8309, p = .0000. The trend of these correlations was

Table 3.2. Correlations Between Age Groups of Preschool Children and the Three Levels of the Group Interaction Scale

Pairs of Variables	Spearman's r	p
2- to 3-year-olds and parallel level (n = 12 groups, 131 children)	−.8805	.0000
3- to 4-year olds and associative level (n = 10 groups, 134 children)	.7139	.0003
4- to 5-year-olds and basic cooperative level (n = 9 groups, 111 children)	.8309	.0000

Note. N = 21 groups of 242 children.

From "Group Profile Studies With Children: Validity Measures and Item Analysis," by M. V. Donohue, 2003, *Occupational Therapy in Mental Health, 19,* p. 13. Copyright © 2003, by Taylor & Francis. Used with permission.

expected, given the results of the study shown in Table 3.2 and Figure 3.1 (Gliner & Morgan, 2000).

Factor and cluster analysis

Building on the relationship between the construct of age and its association with the SP's social participation levels using the first three levels of the SP as a continuous construct, an exploratory factor analysis was undertaken. In the analysis, the component matrix, the pattern matrix, and the structure matrix indicated that the SP had four major components. Looking at the breakdown of the total variance explained, these four components accounted for 85% of the cumulative variance. The basic cooperative behavior items had the highest loadings of the pattern matrix (range = .949 to .720), making up Component 1 of the factor analysis. The associative

behavior items had the next highest loadings (range = −.946 to −.432), making up Component 2. The parallel behavior items (range = .914 to .127) had the next highest loadings, making up Components 3 and 4 (Donohue, 2003; Kim & Mueller, 1978; Saracho, 1993; Spector, 1992; Weinberg & Goldberg, 1990).

The contribution of the basic cooperative behaviors to the variance was large, accounting for 61%. The other three components combined accounted for only 23.8% of the variance: 11.6% for associative behaviors and 12.2% for parallel behaviors. The separateness of these factors is illustrated in the plot of the three levels, indicating discrete clusters in the three-dimensional areas (see Figure 3.2). This result is confirmed by the low correlations of each of the four component factors of the analysis (range = .307 to .451; for the unforced

Figure 3.2. Factor analysis plot of the basic cooperative, associative, and parallel levels.

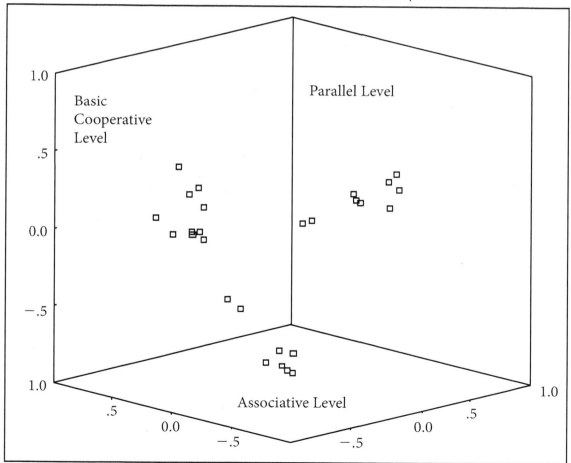

Note. From "Group Profile Studies With Children: Validity Measures and Item Analysis," by M. V. Donohue, 2003, *Occupational Therapy in Mental Health, 19,* p. 13. Copyright © 2003 by Taylor and Francis. Reprinted with permission.

rotation, range = −.382 to −.436). This finding indicates that although the behavioral-level components are distinct, they make up a unidimensional profile (Kim & Mueller, 1978).

Figure 3.2 illustrates the three-dimensional position of the component-level behaviors as they relate to each other in the rotation. The basic cooperative–level items are centered in the left quadrant, the associative-level items are centered in or near the lower quadrant, and the parallel-level items are centered in or near the right quadrant, demonstrating the separation of the three group skill-level concepts within the continuum construct.

In the studies of the longer form of the SP with 15 groups (Donohue, 2005) of preschool children, a statistical cluster analysis was carried out to assess whether scores for the group-level skill behaviors are located together under the clinical or theoretical factors, as would be expected in the construct of progressive social behavior levels. A cluster analysis searches for relationships among the items in a matrix to locate which items are similar (Bernard, 2000) and includes aspects of discriminant analysis, chi-square analysis, and factor analysis (Donohue, 2005).

Two occupational therapy observers examined the factors of parallel, associative, and basic cooperative levels in conjunction with the group process factors of cooperation, norms, roles, communication, activity, power, and attraction. A statistician guided the work of this analysis, which resulted in 21 cells of expected interaction

(7 factors × 3 social participation levels; see Table 3.3; H. Kaplan, personal communication, July 21, 1997).

Table 3.3 shows that the group participation scores for the observers fell into the 21 cells according to theoretical and clinical expectations. For both observers, 21 of 21 cases fell into the expected cells because the social participation scores intersected within the appropriate cluster and variable cells. The work of the two observers was not correlated; however, both of their observations confirmed the expected construct relationships (Donohue, 2005).

Another factor analysis was conducted by Donohue (2005) of the longer version of the SP to plot the four major components of social participation behaviors incorporated into the study. Data from 15 groups of preschool children were entered into this factor analysis in four groupings: The factor loadings for parallel behaviors ranged from −.789 to −.900; for supportive cooperative behaviors, from .841 to .930; for associative behaviors, from .779 to .949; and for basic cooperative behaviors, from .649 to .755 (Donohue, 2005; Kim & Mueller, 1978; Miller, 1989).

Parallel behaviors were the most common although negative in value, which is not unexpected because they do not include interaction and are thus pregrouped. Their nature, conceptually and clinically without participation, has been confirmed statistically. Parallel, supportive cooperative, and associative behaviors were in the high range; however, basic cooperative behaviors were in the moderate range.

Table 3.3. Cluster Analysis and Group Membership of Seven Group Process Factors in Three Social Profile Levels Across Parallel, Associative, and Basic Cooperative Items

Group Level	Group Process Factors						
	Cooperation	Norms	Roles	Communication	Activity	Power	Attraction
Observer 1 (21 variables)							
Parallel	.64	.72	.64	.44	.66	.45	.74
Associative	.81	.70	.59	.60	.45	.57	.48
Basic cooperative	.61	.89	.71	.37	.54	.60	.53
Observer 2 (21 variables)							
Parallel	.65	.68	.88	.64	.64	.53	.48
Associative	.43	.38	.42	.27	.33	.54	.50
Basic cooperative	.56	.52	.43	.43	.46	.44	.41

Note. Adapted from "Social Profile: Assessment of Validity and Reliability With Preschool Children," by M. V. Donohue, 2005, *Canadian Journal of Occupational Therapy, 72,* p. 170. Copyright © 2005, by Sage. Used with permission.

The first factor, parallel behaviors, represented 47.6% of the variance. The other three factors jointly made up 38.7% of the variance of the factor analysis: Supportive cooperative behaviors had 23.5% of the variance; associative behaviors, 10.9% of the variance; and basic cooperative behaviors, only 4.3% of the variance. Both exploratory and confirmatory factor analysis methods and rotations were used and yielded the same four major factors (Donohue, 2005; Kim & Mueller, 1978).

Figure 3.3 illustrates four very separate factors in a three-dimensional plot depiction of rotated space. Despite the clusters' numeric sequence of variance percentage-wise, the supportive cooperative cluster is positioned in the upper-left quadrant, with the basic cooperative cluster below it in the same quadrant. The associative cluster is in the right quadrant, trailing below the basic cooperative cluster, and the parallel cluster is lowest of all in the right quadrant. Together, from left to right, they form an "S" configuration. The

plot clusters were coded from 1 to 4, identifying factor categories corresponding to the conceptual category levels for the purpose of analysis, and emerged in the order shown.

Criterion validity

Parten's (1932) study is the closest criterion for comparison and contrast with the SP. Her study included 6 children, with 60 data points recorded for each child, resulting in 360 data points. Parten separated the children into five preschool age groups ranging from 2 to 4.5 years old. As in studies with the SP (Donohue, 2003, 2005), Parten's data indicated that the largest number of parallel behaviors occur in children ages 2 to 3 years. Likewise, associative behaviors in Parten's study demonstrated trends similar to those in the SP studies, with a gradual increase in associative behaviors in 3- to 4-year-olds' participation.

Finally, Parten's (1932) data showed that cooperative behaviors were highest among children ages 4 to 5

Figure 3.3. Factor analysis of parallel, supportive cooperative, associative, and basic cooperative levels.

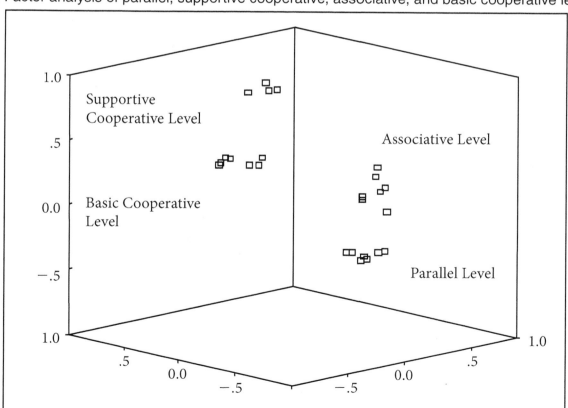

Note. From "Social Profile: Assessment of Validity and Reliability With Preschool Children," by M. V. Donohue, 2005, *Canadian Journal of Occupational Therapy, 72,* p. 171. Copyright © 2005, by Sage. Used with permission.

(Figure 2.1), closely reflecting the groups using the SP, in which cooperative behaviors were highest among 4- to 5-years-olds. Because Parten's study described only summary results, performing an ANOVA to more exactly compare the two studies is not possible. An analysis comparing age-related scores of group participation levels in the two studies resulted in a Spearman correlation coefficient of .85 ($p = .01$, one-tailed). To date, the author has located no study comparable to Lissitz and Samuelsen's (2007) study of the adolescent and adult behavioral concepts in the SP's supportive cooperative and mature levels.

Sensitivity of Social Profile

Research questions regarding the SP's sensitivity led to a study (Donohue, Hanif, & Wu Burns, 2011) examining whether the SP could measure changes in social interaction brought about by participation in occupational therapy activity groups. Thirty psychiatric patients with diagnoses of schizophrenia, bipolar disorder, depression, and obsessive–compulsive disorder at an urban hospital were studied using the SP to rate their social behaviors. They were observed on two occasions, early in their admission to the occupational therapy activity groups and just before discharge, after approximately 30 days of occupational therapy and unit services, and their social behaviors were rated using the SP.

Criteria for admission to the study included being in a group and displaying some potential for improvement. Two therapists in two groups from two similar units led the patients in activities such as making wooden crafts, for example, a stool, box, and coat rack; meal planning; cooking; listening to music; patient government; weekend planning; grooming; stress management; assertiveness training; movement; and life skills.

A t test was carried out on this paired-data sample (SPSS, Version 17; SPSS, Inc., Chicago). Because improvement in SP scores was expected, the test was one tailed, with the level of significance set at .05. With a degree of freedom of 29, the critical one-tailed t was 1.699. The mean for the SP pretest scores was 62.1666; for the posttest scores, it was 84.333, with the higher score indicating improvement. The observed one-tailed t was 4.750, higher than the critical t, thus appearing to be significantly different (SPSS, 2008). To test the statistical power of this study's t test of means, a G*Power test (Buchner, Erdfelder, & Faul, 1997; Dusseldorf University, 2010) was conducted on the difference between the dependent-matched pretest and posttest scores; it yielded a power of 0.835357, indicating an effect size of 0.5. Social scientists view effect sizes from 0.3 to 0.5 as moderate effect size, indicating that a t test has moderately important or meaningful power (Buchner et al., 1997; MEERA, 2007). Figure 3.4 illustrates the

Figure 3.4. Pre- and posttest scores of 30 psychiatric patients after 30 days of occupational therapy group treatment.

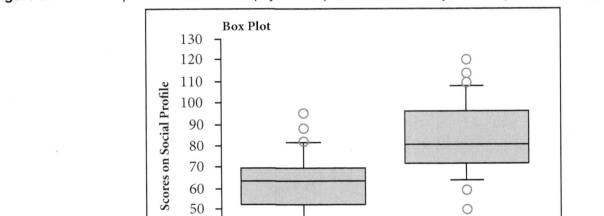

Note. From "An Exploratory Study of Social Participation in Occupational Therapy Groups," by M. V. Donohue, H. Hanif, and L. Wu Berns, 2011, *Mental Health Special Interest Section Quarterly, 34*(3), p. 3. Copyright © 2011, by the American Occupational Therapy Association. Reprinted with permission.

pretest and posttest scores on the SP's continuum of scores (Polit & Hungler, 1995; Stein, Rice, & Cutler, 2013).

Donohue and colleagues' study (2011) illustrates that the SP is sensitive enough to detect differences between social participation scores observed in occupational therapy activity groups over a 1-month time span. It also may indicate that occupational therapy groups, with their activities and discussion of interaction, goals, and activity participation, have the potential to aid patients in recovery from psychiatric illness. In addition to occupational therapy interventions, the psychiatric patients on these units were receiving treatment from psychiatrists, psychologists, social workers, and psychiatric nurses. The combination of these five professions' interventions is what was measured in this study (Donohue et al., 2011).

The results of the Spearman correlation, ANOVA, item analysis, cluster and factor analyses, and *t* test revealed that the relationships among the SP's five levels of social participation are separate and do progress along a rank ordered continuum as people grow older. These relationships strongly suggest that the concepts of the SP form a developmental construct of social interaction or cooperation and confirm their use by educators, psychologists, and occupational therapists.

The association of age as a construct with the five levels of social participation enables one to view the SP as a continuum. The results of these studies (Donohue, 2003, 2005, 2006; Donohue et al., 2011) validate clinical and theoretical hypotheses about age and group developmental levels of social performance, indicating that a graded scale such as the SP is able to measure a range of score levels. The *t*-test sensitivity study indicated that the SP can detect differences in behavioral performances through observation of social participation in activity groups.

Reliability Studies

Reliability studies carried out for the SP included a study of internal consistency reliability of items, interrater reliability of the long form of the SP, interrater reliability of the short form of the SP, and a pilot study of test–retest reliability.

Internal Consistency Reliability of Items

The discussion of internal consistency reliability of the items of the short form of the SP was placed in the "Analysis of Items' Internal Consistency Reliability" section at the opening of this chapter to indicate how the SP was initially developed and researched.

Interrater Reliability of the Social Profile: Long Form

In a study of 15 preschool groups (Donohue, 2005), two observers used the long form of the SP to observe 187 children typically developing in both age-specific and mixed-age groups during free play. The two observers were psychosocial occupational therapy clinicians with years of activity group leadership experience and had assisted in developing the long version of SP.

An intraclass correlation coefficient (ICC; Shrout & Fleiss, 1979; Yaffee, 1998) and Spearman rank order correlation coefficients were used to examine interrater reliability with nonparametric numbers of participants because groups were analyzed as units. Table 3.4 presents the rating scores of the two observers on parallel-, associative-, and basic cooperative–level behaviors. As can be seen, both parallel and basic cooperative behavior scores of the two raters correlated at highly significant levels ($p < .05$ or $p < .01$). The level of agreement between parallel-level scores was high, with correlations ranging from $r = .712$ to $.902$ ($p < .01$). The level of agreement between basic cooperative–level scores was more moderate, with correlations ranging from $r = .575$ ($p < .05$) to $.798$ ($p < .000$). The specific ICC used in this study was selected in consultation with a statistical research and computer consultant (F. Lopresti, personal communication, November 21, 2001; Donohue, 2005; Shrout & Fleiss, 1979; Yaffee, 1998; see Table 3.4).

In another comparison of the two observers' ratings, the ICC (the average of the 7 variables' correlation for interrater reliability) was .88 ($p < .001$). Although significance is not as relevant as level of agreement, .88 is a good level of interrater reliability across seven abstract, psychosocial variables.

Interrater Reliability of the Social Profile: Short Form

Further studies of interrater reliability for the short form of the SP were carried out in psychosocial psychiatric activity groups varying in cultural background and age (ages 18 to 76 years) in hospital and community settings (Donohue, 2006). Two clinicians paired with two graduate students observed 21 occupational therapy groups on two psychiatric units,

Table 3.4. Spearman Rank Order Correlation Coefficients Comparing Scores of Two Observers Using the Social Profile's Parallel, Associative, and Basic Cooperative–Level Behaviors

	Parallel		Associative		Basic Cooperative	
Factors	r	p	r	p	r	p
Cooperation	.712**	.003	.220	.430	.798**	.000
Norms	.814**	.000	.168	.549	.733**	.002
Roles	.869**	.000	.168	.549	.733**	.002
Communication	.793**	.000	−.054	.848	.600*	.018
Activity involvement	.824**	.000	.214	.443	.653**	.008
Power	.878**	.000	.210	.453	.696**	.004
Attraction/motivation	.902**	.000	−.215	.442	.575*	.025

Note. $N = 187$ preschool children in 15 groups.
$*p < .05.$ $**p < .01.$
From "Social Profile: Assessment of Validity and Reliability With Preschool Children," by M. V. Donohue, 2005, *Canadian Journal of Occupational Therapy, 72,* p. 172. Copyright © 2005, by Sage. Used with permission.

with three types of groups: (1) general, (2) geriatric, and (3) substance abuse treatment. The samples on these units consisted of individuals from a variety of cultural and socioeconomic backgrounds from a two-borough catchment section in a large metropolitan area. The general psychiatric units included patients with schizophrenia, bipolar disorder, depression, and obsessive–compulsive disorder. In addition, 14 community groups were observed by 28 graduate students who used the SP to evaluate 14 preschool, adolescent, and senior center groups in a variety of cultural and socioeconomic areas of a large metropolitan interstate region. In all these settings, the paired observers, clinicians, and students had worked with the groups being observed for 4 to 6 weeks before this study. The observers had also received in-service and seminar training.

The scores of the 32 raters involved in these two studies were examined in pairs using an ICC statistical test (Shrout & Fleiss, 1979), chosen with a

statistical research consultant, designed for analyzing interrater reliability in two matched columns of scores (F. Lopresti, personal communication, November 21, 2001; Shrout & Fleiss, 1979).

The ICC reliability scores for the preschool and senior center groups resulted in $\alpha = .8813$; the studies of psychiatric groups resulted in $\alpha = .8028$. Because the focus of these studies was the correlation of the raters' observations, the data from the two studies were combined, resulting in analysis of 35 sessions with 70 completed SPs. The ICC analysis resulted in $\alpha = .8359$, which is considered moderately high, a good level for psychosocial behaviors of an abstract nature (see Table 3.5; Donohue, 2005, 2006). By examining the SP's profile page, group leaders such as psychologists, social workers, teachers, and psychosocial occupational therapists can obtain a clearer understanding of the level of social participation of activity groups and individuals in those groups (Donohue, 2005, 2006).

Table 3.5. Social Profile Interrater Reliability Studies of Community and Clinical Activity Groups

Observer		Setting	Observation Totals
Type	No. of Pairs or Groups	Type	No. of Profiles or Sessions
Graduate students	28/14	Community-based: preschools, senior centers	28/14
Clinicians and graduate students	4/2	Hospital-based: general and geriatric unit substance abuse unit	42/21
Total	**32/16**		**70/35**

Note. From "Interrater Reliability of the Social Profile: Assessment of Community and Psychiatric Group Participation," by M. V. Donohue, 2006, *Australian Occupational Therapy Journal, 54,* p. 5. Copyright © 2006, by John Wiley and Sons. Reprinted with permission.

Test–Retest Reliability

A pilot study of test–retest reliability using videotapes of activity groups of children and adults was carried out with 20 graduate students who received training in using the SP as an observation tool (Donohue, 2010b). The retest took place approximately 4 weeks after the initial test. The results indicated a reliability-level correlation of $r = .75$, which is adequate for a social behavioral tool (Stein, Rice, & Cutler, 2013). Future reliability studies are planned that will incorporate additional training in the understanding and use of the SP.

Summary of Reliability Studies

To date, the consistency of observations for interrater and test–retest reliability is adequate for studies of children and individual adults in groups and with the group as a whole. Member-checking observations with participants in the studies could reassure investigators of the accuracy of their perceptions of interactive behaviors in social activities and roles.

Summary

Although the studies presented in this chapter were adequate in size, they were not large.

However, no study has disputed the theoretical basis and clinical observations of therapists and educators in their perceptions of the sequence of developmental levels of social participation in groups (Mosey, 1986; Parten, 1932). Furthermore, the studies of older adults indicated that social interaction skills are sustained across the life span and are used appropriately in specific situations (Donohue, 2006). These studies also demonstrated the SP's value as an instrument that is sensitive enough to measure various levels of participation in activity group interactions (American Educational Research Association, American Psychological Association, & National Council on Measurement in Education, 1992; Donohue et al., 2011).

CHAPTER 4

Group Cases: Ratings and Interpretations

The Social Profile (SP) may be used to rate groups as groups in individual sessions or across several sessions by averaging the social and activity behaviors. The SP also may be used to observe and rate an individual's social and activity participation within a group (Donohue, 2003, 2005, 2006; Donohue, Hanif, & Wu Berns, 2011), which allows the therapist to provide a more specific treatment plan for discharge. This plan is especially necessary when group participants rotate into and out of groups for treatment and, as a result, a stable group never remains intact over time at a given level of interaction. In studies of group efficacy, measuring individual behaviors may be needed to follow progress or improvement over time (Bellack, Mueser, Gingerich, & Agresta, 1997; Raphael-Greenfield et al., 2011).

On other occasions, when a group membership remains permanent during an adequately long period of treatment, the group may be rated as a unit for the purposes of outcome studies looking at treatment consequences. While making these ratings, the observer should focus on the majority of the group members and not deviate or be distracted by members with outlier behaviors whose functioning is on the periphery of the group as a whole (Yalom & Leszcz, 2005).

This chapter explains the process of scoring the SP, then provides examples of ratings on the SP forms in a series of cases of various groups, including both typically developing children and adolescents and also adults and groups who need therapeutic intervention. These cases are sequenced developmentally across a continuum of groups, ranging from those mostly at the parallel stage to those mostly at the supportive cooperative and mature stages to assist in interpretation for the administrator.

Scoring

The process of scoring the SP consists of first rating the 39 items of the Adult version or the 32 items of the Children's version using a Likert scale, with 0 = *never,* 1 = *rarely,* 2 = *sometimes,* 3 = *frequently,* 4 = *almost always,* and 5 = *always.* Scoring is done for the following three pages:

- *Topic 1:* Activity participation
- *Topic 2:* Social interaction
- *Topic 3:* Group membership and roles.

To assist the rater, a global question introduces each of the three topics:

- *Topic 1:* How do the activities influence group interaction?
- *Topic 2:* How do group members interact with each other?
- *Topic 3:* Do members feel they belong in the group?

In considering the Likert scores, the rater may examine the group's social and activity interaction during either a single session or across several sessions. If the rater perceives that the group is likely to emphasize activity at the parallel or associative levels of social and activity group participation, the recommendation is to begin by rating those two levels of function. If the rater assesses the group's major performance level as being in the cooperative or mature ranges, the rater is suggested to begin by rating those levels of function. However, reading or reviewing all levels, in addition to the parts of the SP that are immediately relevant, is important in making a thorough assessment.

The parallel group is an aggregate with some awareness of other group members and performs activities relatively independently of each other. When members begin to associate with each other for brief periods of time, they are moving to the associative level of group participation.

In determining a Likert rating for each group level, the rater can average a score across the two to five items describing that level's behaviors. Sometimes a decimal may be used, for example, 2.5, if the rater is deliberating between a Likert score of 2 or 3. (See sample cases provided at the end of this chapter.)

Rationale for Continuum

Because social skills are most frequently manifested across levels of group function, group members should generally exhibit a spectrum of behaviors within and across several levels, which is why the SP is structured and rated as a profile. For example, group members may emphasize behaviors at a level such as basic cooperative and continue to exhibit behaviors achieved at the associative level. Simultaneously, the group members may be making an effort to engage each other at the supportive cooperative level and may manifest some behaviors at this level with lower Likert scale ratings (Cohen, Swerdlik, & Philips, 1995; see the SP's Scoring Instructions).

Raters should incorporate ratings at various levels when a group performs an activity at the associative or basic cooperative levels of participation and then has a reflective discussion at the end of the activity in which some supportive cooperative behaviors are manifested. Raters should bear in mind whether the group functioned independently at a supportive cooperative level or relied on the leader's guidance, in which case the Likert ratings should not be high.

Also note that the supportive cooperative behaviors are accompanied by or consist with a conscious display of emotion. This level of group participation highlights the enjoyment of being with others for its own sake, with the performance and achievement of the task perceived as a secondary accomplishment. Camaraderie is uppermost at this group level. When such a group moves on to emphasize the task as much as the feelings of its members, it is then at the mature level (Dildine, 1972).

Judgment Expertise

Raters should use their judgment to determine whether to incorporate ratings for earlier levels that were achieved and consolidated in a previous period of social skill development, except those for the parallel level when groups manifest much higher levels of interactive performance. In that instance, the parallel level can be scored as 0, indicating that the group is not at that level but beyond it.

Rating social skill levels is not a hard science. Ratings are somewhat relative, reflecting the perceptions of the observer. However, those inexperienced in group observations are recommended to test their ratings through discussion with more seasoned activity group process leaders or discussion with peers to validate the reliability of their ratings and prevent extreme deviations in observation ratings (see Chapter 2).

New group leaders also are advised to improve their expertise by practicing observing groups using the Social Profile Observation Sheet (Exhibit 4.1), identifying the social group behaviors of cooperation, norms, roles, communication, activity behavior, power–leadership, and motivation–attraction. Taking notes on this sheet during or after a group can facilitate more accurate use of the Likert ratings within group levels on the SP. (This sheet can also be found on the flash drive included with this manual.)

Summary Sheet

Transfer the average Likert ratings from the last column of each of the three topic pages to the summary sheet. Then write the average for each of the five social group performance levels in the summary average column. The summary scores then may be averaged for research purposes, if desired, but doing so removes the profile effect for the group's rating.

Graph of the Social Profile

Plot the numbers from the summary sheet on the graph on the last page, indicating the points for activity participation, social interaction, and group membership across the five functional levels (parallel, associative, basic cooperative, supportive cooperative, and mature). Then connect these points to see the group's pattern or profile during a given session or time period of sessions.

Exhibit 4.1. Social Profile Observation Sheet for Ratings of Factors of Group Participation

Observe group for 30 minutes. Take notes on this sheet after group observation. A single behavior may be recorded in several of the areas.

Cooperation:

_____

_____

_____

Norms:

_____

_____

_____

Roles:

_____

_____

_____

Communication:

_____

_____

_____

Activity behaviors:

_____

_____

_____

Power and leadership:

_____

_____

_____

Motivation and attraction:

_____

_____

_____

Goals:

_____

_____

_____

Group Cases

The following case examples are arranged in group-level order from parallel to associative to basic cooperative to supportive cooperative to mature; they are related to level of participation, not age. The cases' scores extend across group participation levels.

Reading all 14 cases and their ratings is helpful to compare the assessment of these behaviors and their levels. Some raters may prefer to score the item ratings with greater distinction and detail than presented here, which is acceptable because social group behaviors can have various interpretations, which may average out to be the same as those presented here. Case Example 4.1 is easy to evaluate, and the summary sheet and graph are filled in to demonstrate how to use them. For the subsequent 13 cases, only the case description, three SP rating pages, and interpretations are presented.

Case Example 4.1. Jon, a 5-Year-Old Child in a Preschool Playgroup

Jon, a 5-year-old boy, participates in a preschool playgroup and is assessed in a free-play setting. He uses a play cell phone to call his friend in the group to ask him to help build a fort out of boxes. His initial outreach is dyadic in nature and is a brief association. The friend agrees, and they soon attract other boys who want to be a part of this project, which looks like fun.

They spend about 15 minutes building the fort and putting flags on it. Jon shares leadership with others and is a major leader of the activity, making many suggestions to the other boys. The boys decide to dress up as pirates, using clothing from the costume trunk in the room. For about 20 minutes, they use the fort as a base to "invade" other parts of the larger group, pretending to use sticks as swords. These activities are longer than those found in an associative group, where joint interaction may last 10 minutes. Jon and the others begin to practice problem solving how to play together with regard to whose suggestions to listen to. They end their activity at an appropriate stopping place.

Jon was able to ask others for assistance in building the fort and gave some assistance in finding the pirates' swords. Jon appears to understand both associative and basic cooperative group rules. Jon and the others began to express ideas for their imaginary play and demonstrated that they could take turns in leader, member, talker, and listener roles. Jon acts as though he has a right to be a group member and leader.

The parallel behaviors in all SP three topics are not observed during this activity. Jon and his friends find the activity more attractive than their relationships, placing them at the basic cooperative level, not at the supportive cooperative level. For Jon and the others, the choice of the activity was motivated by some self-interest. Jon could state his intentions of building a fort and agreed to dressing up as pirates. Jon's goals are matched by his socially acceptable actions (Borg & Bruce, 1991; Case-Smith & Archer, 2008; Crick & Dodge, 1994).

These behaviors are rated for the three topics of activity participation, social interaction, and group membership and roles using Likert scale ratings, which are then totaled; their average is put in the average column. These numbers are next transferred to the Summary Sheet. (*Note.* If no behaviors are manifested at a given level, it is not necessary to write in zeros.)

Case Example 4.1. Jon, a 5-Year-Old Child in a Preschool Playgroup

Name of Group/Child: 5-year-old boy, Jon
Activities: Talks on cell phone, builds fort with boxes, dresses up and plays make believe

Assessment of Activity Participation, Social Interaction, and Membership Roles in a Group

Purpose: The Social Profile (SP) was created to assess group-level functioning during activities. Data from the SP organize a group's developmental and functional levels with a standard numerical coding system.

Three Levels of Group Participation

Parallel. Group members play, move, or work side by side but do not interact with each other.
Associative. Group members approach each other briefly in verbal and nonverbal interactions during play, activity, or work.
Basic cooperative. Group members jointly select, implement, and execute longer play, activity, or work tasks for reasons of mutual self-interest in the goal, project, or fellow members.

Directions: On the basis of your observations of the interactions, please circle the number from 0 to 5 that most clearly describes how often the behavior occurred. Think also about the percentage of time the behaviors are at the parallel, associative, or basic cooperative level. (See **boldface** numbers below.)

Topic 1: Activity participation: Jon talks with one other boy by phone, asking to build a fort together with boxes. Other boys ask to join and then dress up and play pirates for 20 minutes.
How do the activities influence the children's group interactions?

0 = *Never*　　　　1 = *Rarely*　　　　2 = *Sometimes*　　　　3 = *Frequently*　　　　4 = *Almost always*　　　　5 = *Always*

Level	Item Description	Score	Average
Parallel	The activities provide 1. Only little sharing of activity with group members. 2. Only familiar activities that encourage performance of the activity, not group interaction.	0 1 2 3 4 5 0 1 2 3 4 5	1
Associative	The activities include 3. Engagement in short-term activities. 4. Joining in shareable activities with group members. 5. Enjoyment of activities between group members.	0 1 2 3 4 5 0 1 2 3 4 5 0 1 2 3 4 5	3.6
Basic Cooperative	The activities focus on 6. Longer, more complex activities. 7. The reflection of group goals and acceptable actions. 8. Completion of activities. 9. Opportunities to begin group problem solving.	0 1 2 3 4 5 0 1 2 3 4 5 0 1 2 3 4 5 0 1 2 3 4 5	3.8

Topic 2: Social interaction: How do the children in the group interact with each other?

0 = *Never*　　　　1 = *Rarely*　　　　2 = *Sometimes*　　　　3 = *Frequently*　　　　4 = *Almost always*　　　　5 = *Always*

Level	Item Description	Score	Average
Parallel	Members interact 10. Very little with other children. 11. With minimal mutual stimulation or awareness. 12. With awareness of group membership rules. 13. Minimal verbal or nonverbal interaction among group members.	0 1 2 3 4 5 0 1 2 3 4 5 0 1 2 3 4 5 0 1 2 3 4 5	0
Associative	Members have been observed 14. Seeking activity assistance from others. 15. Giving concrete assistance willingly. 16. Understanding give and take in associative rules.	0 1 2 3 4 5 0 1 2 3 4 5 0 1 2 3 4 5	3.8
Basic Cooperative	Members interact by 17. Beginning to express ideas and meet needs of others. 18. Experimenting with group member roles (e.g., talker, initiator, listener). 19. Acting as though they have a right to be group members. 20. Respecting others' rights and basic cooperative rules.	0 1 2 3 4 5 0 1 2 3 4 5 0 1 2 3 4 5 0 1 2 3 4 5	3.8

Topic 3: Group membership and roles: Do the children feel they belong in the group?

0 = Never   1 = Rarely   2 = Sometimes   3 = Frequently   4 = Almost always   5 = Always

Level	Item Description	Score	Average
Parallel	**Members** 21. Appear to trust leaders and others; follow directions with leader's prompting. 22. Are comfortable participating in activities in the presence of others without interaction.	0 **1** 2 3 4 5 0 **1** 2 3 4 5	1.5
Associative	**Members** 23. Begin to interact with some cooperation and competition. 24. Emphasize performance of activities over relationships.	0 1 2 **3** 4 5 0 1 2 **3** 4 5	3
Basic Cooperative	**Members** 25. Activity motivated by some self-interest. 26. Can identify and meet group goals with socially acceptable actions.	0 1 2 3 **4** 5 0 1 2 3 **4** 5	4

Social Profile Summary Sheet

Individual or Group Name:

Social Activity: Talks on cell phone, builds fort with boxes, dresses up as pirate

Directions: Transfer the average scores for each level from each of the three sections of the SP to the appropriate box below. In the summary column, average each level's average. You may average the summaries if the result appears to be clinically or educationally meaningful. On the next page, graph the results of the Likert scores within each level to obtain a profile of the group's social participation during activity interaction. (*Note.* Averages were rounded down to avoid numeric inflation.)

Level	Topic 1. Activity Participation	Topic 2. Social Interaction	Topic 3. Group Membership	Summary Average of Topics 1, 2, and 3
Basic Cooperative	3.8	3.8	4.0	3.86
Associative	3.6	3.8	3.0	3.46
Parallel	1.0	0	1.0	0.6

If meaningful, average of summaries: 2.64

Interpretation:

These averages may appear to be low for Jon, but he and the group did not carry on the activity from 1 day to another (e.g., they did not build the fort on 1 day and play pirates the next day). As children move beyond preschool, they expand their behaviors and performance on the three topics and three levels, typically consolidating gains for the basic cooperative level during childhood up to age 10. They also carry on longer tasks over days and weeks at a time. Jon has solid associative and basic cooperative behaviors and skills, with a lower score in parallel behaviors, which is appropriate for his age. His profile is slightly skewed toward the high end, at a moderate level of performance. Observation of Jon would be recommended during future groups to do a composite profile by "homogenizing" his performance mentally across sessions, then using the Likert scale ratings to create a composite observational picture of his participation across a number of activities and with several children.

Composite Graph: Activity Participation, Social Interaction, and Group Membership

Directions: Plot the numbers from the summary sheet on the graph below, and connect points in a line graph. You may plot the graph horizontally or vertically.

Level		Activity Participation	Social Interaction	Group Membership
Basic Cooperative	5			
	4			4.0
	3	3.8	3.8	
	2			
	1			
	0			
Associative	5			
	4			
	3	3.6	3.8	3.0
	2			
	1			
	0			
Parallel	5			
	4			
	3			
	2			
	1	1.0	0	1.0
	0		0	

Social Profile group cases illustrating parallel to mature levels of participation:

4.2. 2-Year-Old Free-Play Group
4.3. Adult Movement to Music Group
4.4. 3.5-Year-Old Free-Play Group
4.5. 5-Year-Old Free-Play Group
4.6. Psychiatric Group of Adults With Minimum-Challenge Activities
4.7. Adult Psychiatric Inpatient Grooming Group
4.8. Psychiatric Inpatient Adolescent Classroom Group
4.9. Psychiatric Inpatient-Unit Goal-Setting Group
4.10. Psychiatric Inpatient Drug Abuse Prevention-of-Relapse Group
4.11. Adolescent Basketball Game in School Courtyard
4.12. Adult Psychiatric Problem-Solving Group
4.13. High School Dance Decorating Committee Group
4.14. Community Senior Reminiscence Group.

Reading the group cases in this order provides readers the opportunity to see how a variety of activities can be modified or designed to achieve a particular level of group interaction (Aureli & Colecchia, 1996; Bales, 1950; Bar-On, Maree, & Elias, 2007; Bellack et al., 1997; Kam, Greenberg, & Kusche, 2004; Kanas, 1966; Salo-Chydenius, 1996; Tanta, Deitz, White, & Billingsley, 2005).

Case Example 4.2. 2-Year-Old Free-Play Group

Setting: At free play with a variety of toys and supplies, including phones, xylophone, baby carriage, rocker, boat, kitchen corner, shopping cart, scooters, paints, sand table, blocks, Legos, markers, paper plates, construction paper on table with chairs, slide, playhouse.

Activities: Pretend to talk on phone for 30 seconds, gluing, painting, drawing, playing xylophone and drum, drinking juice, pushing strollers alone or side by side, pouring sand at sand table, drawing on floor, hammering on table, building tower with blocks, crawling on slide, looking at books, eating snack at table.

Interaction: Children talking very little to others, sounds of babbling, cooing, noises of toys, humming, singing with music; children frequently talk to teacher. There is some unintelligible baby talk to themselves. Children mostly play by themselves.

Statements: "I want my mommy." "I need that." "That's mine." "Play it right." "Come here." "Look." To teacher: "I want to give you a hug." "I want to go home." "Here" (hands something). Holds doll alone; "Hi, can I hold baby?"

One throws water across table at another; pat, tap, and shake sand in containers; some parallel coloring with markers at table; one points at others; one pokes another child; two hammer together on table; three build a tower together then fight over it; they mostly play by themselves; they ride alone on scooters and cars

Some children are fighting over using the stroller, some sharing in the kitchen, watching others, daydreaming; sharing is minimal, many play alone; but have some tolerance for sharing, the teacher tells them how to take turns, brief involvement with others; three kids laugh in playhouse, two kids in playhouse scream and clap for 2 seconds.

(See Social Profile Form for Case Example 4.2.)

Interpretation of Profile Ratings: This group barely has a profile, because only two of the three topics are scored on the form at more than one level (parallel and associative), and at the second level scored, the rating is only *1* or *rarely* for the associative level, which is typically where most 2-year-olds are in their participation or interaction skills.

Case Example 4.2. 2-Year-Old Free-Play Group

Topic 1: Activity participation: How do the activities influence the children's group interactions?

0 = *Never*   1 = *Rarely*   2 = *Sometimes*   3 = *Frequently*   4 = *Almost always*   5 = *Always*

Level	Item Description	Score	Average
Parallel	**The activities provide**		4
	1. Only little sharing of activity with group members.	0 1 2 3 4 5	
	2. Only familiar activities that encourage performance of the activity, not group interaction.	0 1 2 3 4 5	
Associative	**The activities include**		1
	3. Engagement in short-term activities.	0 1 2 3 4 5	
	4. Joining in shareable activities with group members.	0 1 2 3 4 5	
	5. Enjoyment of activities between group members.	0 1 2 3 4 5	
Basic Cooperative	**The activities focus on**		
	6. Longer, more complex activities.	0 1 2 3 4 5	
	7. The reflection of group goals and acceptable actions.	0 1 2 3 4 5	
	8. Completion of activities.	0 1 2 3 4 5	
	9. Opportunities to begin group problem solving.	0 1 2 3 4 5	

Topic 2: Social interaction: How do children in the group interact with each other?

0 = *Never* 1 = *Rarely* 2 = *Sometimes* 3 = *Frequently* 4 = *Almost always* 5 = *Always*

Level	Item Description	Score	Average
Parallel	**Members interact**		3
	10. Very little with other people.	0 1 2 3 4 5	
	11. With minimal mutual stimulation or awareness.	0 1 2 3 4 5	
	12. With observance of parallel group rules.	0 1 2 3 4 5	
	13. Minimal verbal or nonverbal exchange among group members.	0 1 2 3 4 5	
Associative	**Members have been observed**		1
	14. Seeking activity assistance from others.	0 1 2 3 4 5	
	15. Giving concrete assistance willingly.	0 1 2 3 4 5	
	16. Understanding give and take in associative rules.	0 1 2 3 4 5	
Basic Cooperative	**Members interact by**		
	17. Beginning to express ideas and meet needs of others.	0 1 2 3 4 5	
	18. Experimenting with group member roles (i.e., talker, initiator, listener).	0 1 2 3 4 5	
	19. Acting as though they have a right to be group members.	0 1 2 3 4 5	
	20. Respecting others' rights and basic cooperative rules.	0 1 2 3 4 5	

Topic 3: Group membership and roles: Do children feel they belong in the group?

0 = *Never* 1 = *Rarely* 2 = *Sometimes* 3 = *Frequently* 4 = *Almost always* 5 = *Always*

Level	Item Description	Score	Average
Parallel	**Members**		4
	21. Appear to trust leaders and others; follow directions with leader's prompting.	0 1 2 3 4 5	
	22. Comfortable participating in activities in the presence of others.	0 1 2 3 4 5	
Associative	**Members**		
	23. Begin to interact with some cooperation and competition.	0 1 2 3 4 5	
	24. Emphasize performance of activities over relationships.	0 1 2 3 4 5	
Basic Cooperative	**Members in the group**		
	25. Activity motivated by some self-interest.	0 1 2 3 4 5	
	26. Can identify and meet group goals with socially acceptable actions.	0 1 2 3 4 5	

Case Example 4.3. Adult Movement to Music Group

Setting: Eight chairs in a circle. Group's music of choice playing.

Activities: Without talking, members are moving to music and following the motions and movements of the group leader. Later, members move by taking turns as leaders with others following.

The leader initially sets the pace and movement with the group all seated. Then members take turns leading with their own creative movements.

Next, members move to music while standing, first with the leader guiding the group, then with the members taking turns as leaders.

(Continued)

Case Example 4.3. Adult Movement to Music Group *(cont.)*

At the end of the activity, the leader asks how the group liked the movement, the music, being led, and taking leadership. The members share their opinions as to their preferences for various aspects of the activity.

Interaction: Members stand next to each other, following the leader without any interaction, until the members take turns being leader. At the end of the group, members discuss participation in the group.

During the discussion portion, the members express their opinions to each other and to the leader. Preferences expressed regarding movement and music were not emotional. The activity did not evoke an emotional response in group members.

(See Social Profile Form for Case Example 4.3.)

Interpretation of Profile Ratings: This profile of adults involves a major activity that would largely be at the parallel level if not for the modification of having the members also nonverbally lead the movement to music. This nonverbal participation by the adults incorporates associative behaviors. The discussion at the end of the group session demonstrates interactive skills at a basic cooperative level; because little emotion was expressed, the behaviors were rated as 0 for the supportive cooperative level.

Case Example 4.3. Adult Movement to Music Group

Topic 1: Activity participation: How do the activities influence group interactions?

0 = Never   1 = Rarely   2 = Sometimes   3 = Frequently   4 = Almost always   5 = Always

Level	Item Description	Score	Average
Parallel	**The activities provide**		3
	1. Only little sharing of activity with group members.	0 1 2 **3** 4 5	
	2. Only familiar activities that encourage performance of the activity, not group interaction.	0 1 2 **3** 4 5	
Associative	**The activities include**		3
	3. Engagement in short-term activities.	0 1 2 **3** 4 5	
	4. Joining in shareable activities with group members.	0 1 2 **3** 4 5	
	5. Enjoyment of activities between group members.	0 1 2 **3** 4 5	
Basic Cooperative	**The activities focus on**		3
	6. Longer, more complex activities.	0 1 2 **3** 4 5	
	7. The reflection of group goals and acceptable actions.	0 1 2 **3** 4 5	
	8. Completion of activities.	0 1 2 **3** 4 5	
	9. Opportunities to begin group problem solving.	0 1 2 **3** 4 5	
Supportive Cooperative	**The activities focus on**		0
	10. Attempts to satisfy others' emotional needs by words or actions.	**0** 1 2 3 4 5	
	11. Attempts to satisfy member's emotional needs by words or actions in addition to participation in the group activity.	**0** 1 2 3 4 5	
	12. Members select the activities.	**0** 1 2 3 4 5	
Mature	**The activities provide**		0
	13. Balance between emotional and performance needs of members.	**0** 1 2 3 4 5	
	14. Usually high-level performance, discussion, or product.	**0** 1 2 3 4 5	

Topic 2: Social interaction: How do group members interact with each other?

0 = Never   1 = Rarely   2 = Sometimes   3 = Frequently   4 = Almost always   5 = Always

Level	Item Description	Score	Average
Parallel	**Members interact**		3
	15. Very little with other people.	0 1 2 **3** 4 5	
	16. With minimal mutual stimulation or awareness.	0 1 2 **3** 4 5	
	17. With observance of parallel group rules.	0 1 2 **3** 4 5	
	18. Minimal verbal or nonverbal exchange among group members.	0 1 2 **3** 4 5	
Associative	**Members have been observed**		4
	19. Seeking activity assistance from others.	0 1 2 3 **4** 5	
	20. Giving concrete assistance willingly.	0 1 2 3 **4** 5	
	21. Understanding give and take in associative rules.	0 1 2 3 **4** 5	
Basic Cooperative	**Members interact by**		3
	22. Beginning to express ideas and meet needs of others.	0 1 2 **3** 4 5	
	23. Experimenting with group member roles (i.e., talker, initiator, listener).	0 1 2 **3** 4 5	
	24. Acting as though they have a right to be group members.	0 1 2 **3** 4 5	
	25. Respecting others' rights and basic cooperative rules.	0 1 2 **3** 4 5	
Supportive Cooperative	**Members have been observed to**		0
	26. Encourage self-expression of feelings in others.	**0** 1 2 3 4 5	
	27. Express positive and negative feelings.	**0** 1 2 3 4 5	
	28. Demonstrate caring about others in the group.	**0** 1 2 3 4 5	
Mature	**Members can**		0
	29. Assume a variety of member and leader roles without prompting.	**0** 1 2 3 4 5	

Topic 3: Group membership and roles: Do members feel they belong in the group?

0 = Never   1 = Rarely   2 = Sometimes   3 = Frequently   4 = Almost always   5 = Always

Level	Item Description	Score	Average
Parallel	**Members**		5
	30. Appear to trust leaders and others; follow directions with leader's prompting.	0 1 2 3 4 **5**	
	31. Are comfortable participating in activities in the presence of others.	0 1 2 3 4 **5**	
Associative	**Members**		4
	32. Begin to interact with some cooperation and competition.	0 1 2 3 **4** 5	
	33. Emphasize performance of activities over relationships.	0 1 2 3 **4** 5	
Basic cooperative	**Members**		3
	34. Activity motivated by some self-interest.	0 1 2 **3** 4 5	
	35. Can identify and meet group goals with socially acceptable actions.	0 1 2 **3** 4 5	
Supportive cooperative	**Members**		0
	36. Enjoy equality and compatibility between members.	**0** 1 2 3 4 5	
	37. Participate in mutual need satisfaction around expression of feelings similar to others.	**0** 1 2 3 4 5	
Mature	**Members**		0
	38. Maintain a balance between activity performance and interaction with group members.	**0** 1 2 3 4 5	
	39. Discuss serious topics (e.g., ethics, politics, health).	**0** 1 2 3 4 5	

Case Example 4.4. 3.5-Year-Old Free-Play Group

Setting: Children are at free play with a variety of toys and supplies. Children play with old clothes and costumes, blocks, toys in the kitchen area, toys in the restaurant area, table and chairs, dishes, toy airplanes, dolls, a pedal car, hammers and pegs, phones, a playhouse, a balance beam and pad, a slide, a bench, a sandbox, and plastic figures. Caregivers were present observing children.

Activities: Playing with blocks, building a tower, playing restaurant, playing with airplanes, dressing up in costumes, making guns out of blocks, tea party, setting table, cooking together, smoking cigarettes, eating ice cream, banging on piano, wrestling, talking on phones, playing house, sliding down slide, parading around the room, playing doctor with back rub, mixing sand in sandbox, crawling on floor, hiding under table.

Interaction: Only one child does a puzzle by himself. Some share blocks. Five children play blocks separately. Then three kids play blocks together. One child uses a car to knock another child's blocks over, and a girl laughs. There is conversation in the restaurant, and one child dressed up to go to the restaurant. A girl puts bread on other child's plate. Three children building a castle play together with it. A girl cries when a boy takes her toy. Another boy hits a girl, and she cries. Two children are sharing ice cream. Two girls bang on piano together. Two girls are wrestling. One child is singing, and a boy and girl hum together. A girl pushes a boy out of "tree house." Several children are talking alone on phones. A boy puts his hand out to ask for a tool. A boy takes a girl by the hand and leads her. Two children play on the floor together under the table. Two girls play together on the balance board. Some children coordinate clean-up. Two girls play dog and master. Some kids cut into the middle of the line to the slide, and two girls act goofy. Then many children follow one girl who starts a parade around the room singing.

Statements: "Don't touch those." "What are you making?" "Help me make this." "What are you doing?" "I've got cigarettes." "You could give me one block." "Mine!" "I have some hamburgers here." "I like to eat bananas" (singing). "No, put it right here." "What letter starts your name?" "I put some sugar in." "I can do that." "I see you, baby." "Now it's my turn." "Here's some tea." "Sit next to me." "My mommy. . . ." "Listen, you guys." "I need a piece." "Ling, ling" (singing). "Okay, I'll give you some." "I got your back" (rubbing back while playing doctor). "Where's the chair?" "I can't open my eyes. My eyes hurt" (to doctor).

(See Social Profile Form for Case Example 4.4.)

Interpretation of Profile Ratings: The composite behaviors of these children display a strong associative level, with some remnants of parallel-level behaviors and some attempts to function at a basic cooperative level.

Case Example 4.4. 3.5-Year-Old Free-Play Group

Topic 1: Activity participation: How do the activities influence group interactions?

0 = *Never*   1 = *Rarely*   2 = *Sometimes*   3 = *Frequently*   4 = *Almost always*   5 = *Always*

Level	Item Description	Score	Average
Parallel	The activities provide		
	1. Only little sharing of activity with group members.	0 1 2 3 4 5	2
	2. Only familiar activities that encourage performance of the activity, not group interaction.	0 1 2 3 4 5	
Associative	The activities include		
	3. Engagement in short-term activities.	0 1 2 3 4 5	4
	4. Joining in shareable activities with group members.	0 1 2 3 4 5	
	5. Enjoyment of activities between group members.	0 1 2 3 4 5	

(Continued)

Level	Item Description	Score	Average
Basic Cooperative	The activities focus on 6. Longer, more complex activities. 7. The reflection of group goals and acceptable actions. 8. Completion of activities. 9. Opportunities to begin group problem solving.	0 1 2 3 4 5 0 1 2 3 4 5 0 1 2 3 4 5 0 1 2 3 4 5	1

Topic 2: Social interaction: How do group members interact with each other?

0 = *Never* 1 = *Rarely* 2 = *Sometimes* 3 = *Frequently* 4 = *Almost always* 5 = *Always*

Level	Item Description	Score	Average
Parallel	Members interact 15. Very little with other people. 16. With minimal mutual stimulation or awareness. 17. With observance of parallel group rules. 18. Minimal verbal or nonverbal exchange among group members.	0 1 2 3 4 5 0 1 2 3 4 5 0 1 2 3 4 5 0 1 2 3 4 5	1
Associative	Members have been observed 19. Seeking activity assistance from others. 20. Giving concrete assistance willingly. 21. Understanding give and take in associative rules.	0 1 2 3 4 5 0 1 2 3 4 5 0 1 2 3 4 5	3
Basic Cooperative	Members interact by 22. Beginning to express ideas and meet needs of others. 23. Experimenting with group member roles (i.e., talker, initiator, listener). 24. Acting as though they have a right to be group members. 25. Respecting others' rights and basic cooperative rules.	0 1 2 3 4 5 0 1 2 3 4 5 0 1 2 3 4 5 0 1 2 3 4 5	2

Topic 3: Group membership and roles: Do members feel they belong in the group?

0 = *Never* 1 = *Rarely* 2 = *Sometimes* 3 = *Frequently* 4 = *Almost always* 5 = *Always*

Level	Item Description	Score	Average
Parallel	Members 30. Appear to trust leaders and others; follow directions with leader's prompting. 31. Are comfortable participating in activities in the presence of others.	0 1 2 3 4 5 0 1 2 3 4 5	2
Associative	Members 32. Begin to interact with some cooperation and competition. 33. Emphasize performance of activities over relationships.	0 1 2 3 4 5 0 1 2 3 4 5	4
Basic Cooperative	Members 34. Activity motivated by some self-interest. 35. Can identify and meet group goals with socially acceptable actions.	0 1 2 3 4 5 0 1 2 3 4 5	1.5

Case Example 4.5. 5-Year-Old Free-Play Group

Setting: Romper room with slide, large balls, rocker for two, playhouse, collage and craft tables, free play in preschool room, boondoggle cord, grassy field near outdoor pool. Teachers' aides observe group.

Activities: Sliding down slide, rocking on rocker, playing tag, jumping and bumping on large balls and bolsters, wrestling, playing house, playing doggy, making yarn and ribbon collages, craft play at tables, eating snack, singing, visiting other tables, fixing hair, pretending to be giraffes, playing with toys and male plastic figures, giving out cookies and crackers, reading games, playing hide-and-seek with subgroups chasing each other, milling around, listening to and commenting on music, reacting to bugs outdoors, group of four going to water fountain outside, eating lunch outdoors, somersaulting.

Interaction: Five kids are on slide, and two fight with large balls. Five kids together on a bench go to slide. Two boys wrestle, and two are in a rocker together. Many children are very excited, with loud dialogue, tossing plastic animals to other children. Whoever has the giraffe is the spokesperson. Three boys are in a side conversation, making many animal sounds—at one point, more so than words. Several kids are teaching each other to read—pointing out words with a pencil, looking at pictures together, evaluating by judging easy and hard words. Several children are apologizing to others when encouraged by teachers. Some kids are laughing during hide and seek.

Statements: Comments on norms emerging through name calling, with an expression of desire to stay out of trouble. Safety concerns and warnings are stated, with questions asking for judgment calls about safety and cooperation.

"Watch out!" "It's my turn to be in the house." "We jump from there." "Watch this." "You know how to do that?" "Stop pushing me." "Get up here." "I put my feet all the way down." "Is that scary?" "That's easy." "Ms. J., watch what I can do." "Watch this, you all." "Want to play doggy?" "Stop jumping on top, you street rat." "I want the supplies." "He took my. . . ." "Get away, he'll throw it at you." "I'm making a girl." "I'm making a design." "What do I do with this?" "I want some . . . " "I'm a cookie monster." "Look how much we have." "Look what I made." "What are you making?" "I'm making a butterfly." "Is my name on that?" "I'm taking this color." "I just want a little kitty." "What do you want?" "Whatever you want." "Look, I'm going to go into the house." "I need green." "Let me read the book." "I can't hear you; talk louder." "Thank you, Tony." "Leave it." "You waste too much; drink it." "Yo-oh." "This is my ring." "Guess again, fat boy, look." "We need you." "C'mon over to this table." "You're going to get me in trouble." "I am a bad guy." "Ah ha, that's a pig." "Want to see a pig, Tony?" "Woo, da, da, da." "Now back to bad-guy world." "I'm going to good-guy world." "One more to go." (Burp) "Excuse me." "I don't want your crackers." "Ouch, stop that." "You smell." "YOU smell." "Look what I see in Disney World." "Can you do this?" "Could I have yellow?" "I have on my bathing suit." "Move! A bug." "I like that song." "I like this part of a dance." "That's my song." "That's my favorite. Me, too." "I'll step on your apple." "Can you do this?" "I don't have my swimsuit on."

(See Social Profile Form for Case Example 4.5.)

Interpretation of Profile Ratings: The group of 5-year-olds scores at a solid associative level, with some manifestation of basic cooperative–level functional behaviors to provide a profile reflecting a continuum for Topics 1 and 2. Under Topic 3, group membership and roles, this age group performs many activities at the basic cooperative level; motivated by some self-interest, they rarely to sometimes meet the whole group's goals.

Case Example 4.5. 5-Year-Old Free-Play Group

Topic 1: Activity participation: How do the activities influence the children's group interactions?

0 = Never   1 = Rarely   2 = Sometimes   3 = Frequently   4 = Almost always   5 = Always

Level	Item Description	Score	Average
Parallel	**The activities provide**		1
	1. Only little sharing of activity with group members.	0 1 2 3 4 5	
	2. Only familiar activities that encourage performance of the activity, not group interaction.	0 1 2 3 4 5	
Associative	**The activities include**		4
	3. Engagement in short-term activities.	0 1 2 3 4 5	
	4. Joining in shareable activities with group members.	0 1 2 3 4 5	
	5. Enjoyment of activities between group members.	0 1 2 3 4 5	
Basic Cooperative	**The activities focus on**		3
	6. Longer, more complex activities.	0 1 2 3 4 5	
	7. The reflection of group goals and acceptable actions.	0 1 2 3 4 5	
	8. Completion of activities.	0 1 2 3 4 5	
	9. Opportunities to begin group problem solving.	0 1 2 3 4 5	

Topic 2: Social interaction: How do group members interact with each other?

0 = Never   1 = Rarely   2 = Sometimes   3 = Frequently   4 = Almost always   5 = Always

Level	Item Description	Score	Average
Parallel	**Members interact**		1
	10. Very little with other people.	0 1 2 3 4 5	
	11. With minimal mutual stimulation or awareness	0 1 2 3 4 5	
	12. With observance of parallel group rules.	0 1 2 3 4 5	
	13. Minimal verbal or nonverbal exchange among group members.	0 1 2 3 4 5	
Associative	**Members have been observed**		4
	14. Seeking activity assistance from others.	0 1 2 3 4 5	
	15. Giving concrete assistance willingly.	0 1 2 3 4 5	
	16. Understanding give and take in associative rules.	0 1 2 3 4 5	
Basic Cooperative	**Members interact by**		3
	17. Beginning to express ideas and meet needs of others.	0 1 2 3 4 5	
	18. Experimenting with group member roles (i.e., talker, initiator, listener).	0 1 2 3 4 5	
	19. Acting as though they have a right to be group members.	0 1 2 3 4 5	
	20. Respecting others' rights and basic cooperative rules.	0 1 2 3 4 5	

Topic 3: Group membership and roles: Do members feel they belong in the group?

0 = Never   *1 = Rarely*   *2 = Sometimes*   *3 = Frequently*   *4 = Almost always*   *5 = Always*

Level	Item Description	Score	Average
Parallel	**Members** 21. Appear to trust leaders and others; follow directions with leader's prompting. 22. Are comfortable participating in activities in the presence of others.	0 1 2 3 4 5 0 1 2 3 4 5	1
Associative	**Members** 23. Begin to interact with some cooperation and competition. 24. Emphasize performance of activities over relationships.	0 1 2 3 4 5 0 1 2 3 4 5	4
Basic Cooperative	**Members** 25. Activity motivated by some self-interest. 26. Can identify and meet group goals with socially acceptable actions.	0 1 2 3 4 5 0 1 2 3 4 5	3

Case Example 4.6. Psychiatric Group of Adults With Minimum-Challenge Activities

Setting: Psychiatric inpatient unit room. Music is played for first activity. Chairs are available. This group is leader-directed.

Activities:
- *Follow the leader.* The therapist guides the group in a parade around the room in which each person walks with a hand on the shoulder of the person in front of him or her in time to the music.
- *Pass the shoe.* Chairs are placed in a circle. Each person takes off one shoe, and all shoes are placed on the floor in the middle of the circle. Everyone is told to take a shoe from the center, but not their own. When the therapist says "Begin," each person passes the shoe to the right until receiving his or her own shoe. The first person to obtain his or her own shoe wins and puts it on. The game continues until everyone gets his or her shoe back. The last person to get his or her shoe back loses the game.
- *Celebrating a holiday (or, my favorite lyrics).* The leader asks, "Does anyone know a poem or the words of a song for a holiday? Or would you like to recite or sing your favorite lyrics of a song?" Group members take turns reciting poems or the words of a song.

Interaction:
- During follow the leader, people are lined up in a row, with only the nonverbal interaction of touching the shoulder of the person in front of them.
- During the "pass the shoes" game, group members reach over to other members as they pass the shoes along. They call out when they obtain their own shoe.
- Everyone listens to the poems and lyrics as they are recited. They clap as each person finishes.

Discussion: The group briefly talks about which of the activities they enjoyed and who they were sitting next to. They briefly describe how well the group participated in the activities.

(See Social Profile Form for Case Example 4.6.)

Interpretation of Profile Ratings: This group's activity participation behaviors place it strongly in the associative level of function because, although they are adults, they need guidance in setting up and following activities as a whole group. The spectrum of the group's SP has a short span, yet is not as strong in its Likert scores as other mostly associative activity groups. Although the group respects each other's rights, its members only identify their own preferences, not those of others, and only identify group goals sometimes. This group is rated as spanning the parallel to basic cooperative levels.

Case Example 4.6. Psychiatric Group of Adults With Minimum-Challenge Activities

Topic 1: Activity participation: How do the activities influence group interactions?

0 = *Never*   1 = *Rarely*   2 = *Sometimes*   3 = *Frequently*   4 = *Almost always*   5 = *Always*

Level	Item Description	Score	Average
Parallel	The activities provide		2
	1. Only little sharing of activity with group members.	0 1 2 3 4 5	
	2. Only familiar activities that encourage performance of the activity, not group interaction.	0 1 2 3 4 5	
Associative	The activities include		4
	3. Engagement in short-term activities.	0 1 2 3 4 5	
	4. Joining in shareable activities with group members.	0 1 2 3 4 5	
	5. Enjoyment of activities between group members.	0 1 2 3 4 5	
Basic Cooperative	The activities focus on		2
	6. Longer, more complex activities.	0 1 2 3 4 5	
	7. The reflection of group goals and acceptable actions.	0 1 2 3 4 5	
	8. Completion of activities.	0 1 2 3 4 5	
	9. Opportunities to begin group problem solving.	0 1 2 3 4 5	
Supportive Cooperative	The activities focus on		0
	10. Attempts to satisfy others' emotional needs by words or actions.	0 1 2 3 4 5	
	11. Attempts to satisfy member's emotional needs by words or actions in addition to participation in the group activity.	0 1 2 3 4 5	
	12. Members select the activities.	0 1 2 3 4 5	
Mature	The activities provide		0
	13. Balance between emotional and performance needs of members.	0 1 2 3 4 5	
	14. Usually high-level performance, discussion, or product.	0 1 2 3 4 5	

Topic 2: Social interaction: How do group members interact with each other?

0 = *Never*   1 = *Rarely*   2 = *Sometimes*   3 = *Frequently*   4 = *Almost always*   5 = *Always*

Level	Item Description	Score	Average
Parallel	Members interact		2
	15. Very little with other people.	0 1 2 3 4 5	
	16. With minimal mutual stimulation or awareness.	0 1 2 3 4 5	
	17. With observance of parallel group rules.	0 1 2 3 4 5	
	18. Minimal verbal or nonverbal exchange among group members.	0 1 2 3 4 5	
Associative	Members have been observed		3
	19. Seeking activity assistance from others.	0 1 2 3 4 5	
	20. Giving concrete assistance willingly.	0 1 2 3 4 5	
	21. Understanding give and take in associative rules.	0 1 2 3 4 5	
Basic Cooperative	Members interact by		2.3
	22. Beginning to express ideas and meet needs of others.	0 1 2 3 4 5	
	23. Experimenting with group member roles (e.g., talker, initiator, listener).	0 1 2 3 4 5	
	24. Acting as though they have a right to be group members.	0 1 2 3 4 5	
	25. Respecting others' rights and basic cooperative rules.	0 1 2 3 4 5	

(Continued)

Level	Item Description	Score	Average
Supportive Cooperative	**Members have been observed to** 26. Encourage self-expression of feelings in others. 27. Express positive and negative feelings. 28. Demonstrate caring about others in the group.	0 1 2 3 4 5 0 1 2 3 4 5 0 1 2 3 4 5	0
Mature	**Members can** 29. Assume a variety of member and leader roles without prompting.	0 1 2 3 4 5	0

Topic 3: Group membership and roles: Do members feel they belong in the group?

0 = *Never*   1 = *Rarely*   2 = *Sometimes*   3 = *Frequently*   4 = *Almost always*   5 = *Always*

Level	Item Description	Score	Average
Parallel	**Members** 30. Appear to trust leaders and others; follow directions with leader's prompting. 31. Are comfortable participating in activities in the presence of others.	0 1 2 **3** 4 5 0 1 2 **3** 4 5	3
Associative	**Members** 32. Begin to interact with some cooperation and competition. 33. Emphasize performance of activities over relationships.	0 1 2 3 **4** 5 0 1 2 3 **4** 5	4
Basic Cooperative	**Members** 34. Activity motivated by some self-interest. 35. Can identify and meet group goals with socially acceptable actions.	0 1 **2** 3 4 5 0 1 **2** 3 4 5	2.5
Supportive Cooperative	**Members** 36. Enjoy equality and compatibility between members. 37. Participate in mutual need satisfaction around expression of feelings similar to others.	**0** 1 2 3 4 5 **0** 1 2 3 4 5	0
Mature	**Members** 38. Maintain a balance between activity performance and interaction with group members. 39. Discuss serious topics (e.g., ethics, politics, health).	**0** 1 2 3 4 5 **0** 1 2 3 4 5	0

Case Example 4.7. Adult Psychiatric Inpatient Grooming Group

Setting: An inpatient-unit occupational therapy room with one sink, its basin filled with water for shaving; razors; shaving cream; multiple mirrors; nail files; an assortment of nail polish; nail polish remover; and combs

Activities: Group members (12 men and women) practice putting on shaving cream, shaving, wiping off cream, and giving the razor back to the occupational therapist. Others file nails, clip hangnails, and apply polish for themselves or for others. They comb and arrange hair.

Interaction: Eight patients are at lowest level of function with many acute symptoms and in pajamas or green gowns; four are dressed in day clothes. Twelve group members, two students, one aide, and one therapist are present.

Some group members tell others if they did not correctly apply cream, shave, or wipe off cream. Some barely look in the mirror and have cream left on their faces. Many file nails, some for themselves and others for other group members. Some apply nail polish for themselves, and others apply it for others. Most group members comb their own hair, but some do someone else's hair. Some ask how their hair looks.

(Continued)

Discussion: The therapist asks people to describe how they did in their grooming activity. "What could they do better next time?" There is some discussion, but not everyone participates. A few people are the main speakers. (See Social Profile Form for Case Example 4.7.)

Interpretation of Profile Ratings: Individual members of this group are at various levels of social interaction and activity participation; therefore, their skills and behaviors span three functional levels. Some members assist and care for others in the group by helping out with their grooming, but most individually groom themselves, so their scores are rated between the parallel and basic cooperative levels of interaction.

Case Example 4.7. Adult Psychiatric Inpatient Grooming Group

Topic 1: Activity participation: How do the activities influence group interactions?

0 = *Never*   1 = *Rarely*   2 = *Sometimes*   3 = *Frequently*   4 = *Almost always*   5 = *Always*

Level	Item Description	Score	Average
Parallel	**The activities provide**		3
	1. Only little sharing of activity with group members.	0 1 2 3 4 5	
	2. Only familiar activities that encourage performance of the activity, not group interaction.	0 1 2 3 4 5	
Associative	**The activities include**		2.5
	3. Engagement in short-term activities.	0 1 2 3 4 5	
	4. Joining in shareable activities with group members.	0 1 2 3 4 5	
	5. Enjoyment of activities between group members.	0 1 2 3 4 5	
Basic Cooperative	**The activities focus on**		2
	6. Longer, more complex activities.	0 1 2 3 4 5	
	7. The reflection of group goals and acceptable actions.	0 1 2 3 4 5	
	8. Completion of activities.	0 1 2 3 4 5	
	9. Opportunities to begin group problem solving.	0 1 2 3 4 5	
Supportive Cooperative	**The activities focus on**		0
	10. Attempts to satisfy others' emotional needs by words or actions.	0 1 2 3 4 5	
	11. Attempts to satisfy member's emotional needs by words or actions in addition to participation of the group activity.	0 1 2 3 4 5	
	12. Members select the activities.	0 1 2 3 4 5	
Mature	**The activities provide**		0
	13. Balance between emotional and performance needs of members.	0 1 2 3 4 5	
	14. Usually high-level performance, discussion, or product.	0 1 2 3 4 5	

Topic 2: Social interaction: How do group members interact with each other?

0 = *Never*　　　1 = *Rarely*　　　2 = *Sometimes*　　　3 = *Frequently*　　　4 = *Almost always*　　　5 = *Always*

Level	Item Description	Score	Average
Parallel	**Members interact**		4
	15. Very little with other people.	0 1 2 3 4 **5**	
	16. With minimal mutual stimulation or awareness.	0 1 2 3 **4** 5	
	17. With observance of parallel group rules.	0 1 2 3 **4** 5	
	18. Minimal verbal or nonverbal exchange among group members.	0 1 2 3 **4** 5	
Associative	**Members have been observed**		2
	19. Seeking activity assistance from others.	0 1 **2** 3 4 5	
	20. Giving concrete assistance willingly.	0 1 **2** 3 4 5	
	21. Understanding give and take in associative rules.	0 1 **2** 3 4 5	
Basic Cooperative	**Members interact by**		2.5
	22. Beginning to express ideas and meet needs of others.	0 1 2 **3** 4 5	
	23. Experimenting with group member roles (e.g., talker, initiator, listener).	0 **1** 2 3 4 5	
	24. Acting as though they have a right to be group members.	0 1 2 **3** 4 5	
	25. Respecting others' rights and basic cooperative rules.	0 1 2 **3** 4 5	
Supportive Cooperative	**Members have been observed to**		0
	26. Encourage self-expression of feelings in others.	**0** 1 2 3 4 5	
	27. Express positive and negative feelings.	**0** 1 2 3 4 5	
	28. Demonstrate caring about others in the group.	**0** 1 2 3 4 5	
Mature	**Members can**		0
	29. Assume a variety of member and leader roles without prompting.	**0** 1 2 3 4 5	

Topic 3: Group membership and roles: Do members feel they belong in the group?

0 = *Never*　　　1 = *Rarely*　　　2 = *Sometimes*　　　3 = *Frequently*　　　4 = *Almost always*　　　5 = *Always*

Level	Item Description	Score	Average
Parallel	**Members**		4
	30. Appear to trust leaders and others; follow directions with leader's prompting.	0 1 2 3 **4** 5	
	31. Are comfortable participating in activities in the presence of others.	0 1 2 3 **4** 5	
Associative	**Members**		3
	32. Begin to interact with some cooperation and competition.	0 1 2 **3** 4 5	
	33. Emphasize performance of activities over relationships.	0 1 2 **3** 4 5	
Basic Cooperative	**Members**		2
	34. Activity motivated by some self-interest.	0 1 **2** 3 4 5	
	35. Can identify and meet group goals with socially acceptable actions.	0 1 **2** 3 4 5	
Supportive Cooperative	**Members**		0
	36. Enjoy equality and compatibility between members.	**0** 1 2 3 4 5	
	37. Participate in mutual need satisfaction around expression of feelings similar to others.	**0** 1 2 3 4 5	
Mature	**Members**		0
	38. Maintain a balance between activity performance and interaction with group members.	**0** 1 2 3 4 5	
	39. Discuss serious topics (e.g., ethics, politics, health).	**0** 1 2 3 4 5	

Case Example 4.8. Psychiatric Inpatient Adolescent Classroom Group

Setting: The setting is a small classroom with a blackboard and desks. There are 7 eighth-grade students with social and academic challenges and a variety of cognitive and emotional functional levels.

Activities: The group reads scrambled sentences about the sinking of the Titanic. They decide on the order of the story in a paragraph. The group sequences the scrambled sentences into an orderly paragraph. Each student reads aloud one sentence from the sequence to tell the story they arranged. After the reading, they assess each other's performance and learn how to speak to others in giving feedback.

Interaction: Students stand in a semicircle, sequentially reading one sentence at a time as a logical, cognitive activity, taking turns inserting their sentence at the appropriate time.

(See the Social Profile Form for Case Example 4.7.)

Interpretation of Profile Ratings: Sharable activities are manifested in this group. During the discussion at the end of the group, they assess each other's performance in learning how to speak aloud in the class and by evaluating how they talk to each other. Because this activity is structured, the reading portions of it are performed at an associative level and the discussion portion functions at a basic cooperative level. Group members can follow the classroom rules for joint group story reading, which helps them share the responsibility for telling the story.

Case Example 4.8. Psychiatric Inpatient Adolescent Classroom Group

Topic 1: Activity participation: How do the activities influence group interactions?

0 = *Never*　　1 = *Rarely*　　2 = *Sometimes*　　3 = *Frequently*　　4 = *Almost always*　　5 = *Always*

Level	Item Description	Score	Average
Parallel	**The activities provide**		3
	1. Only little sharing of activity with group members.	0 1 2 3 4 5	
	2. Only familiar activities that encourage performance of the activity, not group interaction.	0 1 2 3 4 5	
Associative	**The activities include**		4
	3. Engagement in short-term activities.	0 1 2 3 4 5	
	4. Joining in shareable activities with group members.	0 1 2 3 4 5	
	5. Enjoyment of activities between group members.	0 1 2 3 4 5	
Basic Cooperative	**The activities focus on**		2
	6. Longer, more complex activities.	0 1 2 3 4 5	
	7. The reflection of group goals and acceptable actions.	0 1 2 3 4 5	
	8. Completion of activities.	0 1 2 3 4 5	
	9. Opportunities to begin group problem solving.	0 1 2 3 4 5	
Supportive Cooperative	**The activities focus on**		0
	10. Attempts to satisfy others' emotional needs by words and actions.	0 1 2 3 4 5	
	11. Attempts to satisfy member's emotional needs by words and actions in addition to participation in the group activity.	0 1 2 3 4 5	
	12. Members select the activities.	0 1 2 3 4 5	
Mature	**The activities provide**		0
	13. Balance between emotional and performance needs of members.	0 1 2 3 4 5	
	14. Usually high-level performance, discussion, or product.	0 1 2 3 4 5	

Topic 2: Social interaction: How do group members interact with each other?

0 = *Never*   1 = *Rarely*   2 = *Sometimes*   3 = *Frequently*   4 = *Almost always*   5 = *Always*

Level	Item Description	Score	Average
Parallel	**Members interact**		3
	15. Very little with other people.	0 1 2 **3** 4 5	
	16. With minimal mutual stimulation or awareness.	0 1 2 **3** 4 5	
	17. With observance of parallel group rules.	0 1 2 **3** 4 5	
	18. Minimal verbal or nonverbal exchange among group members.	0 1 2 **3** 4 5	
Associative	**Members have been observed**		4
	19. Seeking activity assistance from others.	0 1 2 3 **4** 5	
	20. Giving concrete assistance willingly.	0 1 2 3 **4** 5	
	21. Understanding give and take in associative rules.	0 1 2 3 4 **5**	
Basic Cooperative	**Members interact by**		3
	22. Beginning to express ideas and meet needs of others.	0 1 2 **3** 4 5	
	23. Experimenting with group member roles (e.g., talker, initiator, listener).	0 1 **2** 3 4 5	
	24. Acting as though they have a right to be group members.	0 1 2 **3** 4 5	
	25. Respecting others' rights and basic cooperative rules.	0 1 2 3 **4** 5	
Supportive Cooperative	**Members have been observed to**		0
	26. Encourage self-expression of feelings in others.	**0** 1 2 3 4 5	
	27. Express positive and negative feelings.	**0** 1 2 3 4 5	
	28. Demonstrate caring about others in the group.	**0** 1 2 3 4 5	
Mature	**Members can**		0
	29. Assume a variety of member and leader roles without prompting.	**0** 1 2 3 4 5	

Topic 3: Group membership and roles: Do members feel they belong in the group?

0 = *Never*   1 = *Rarely*   2 = *Sometimes*   3 = *Frequently*   4 = *Almost always*   5 = *Always*

Level	Item Description	Score	Average
Parallel	**Members**		3
	30. Appear to trust leaders and others; follow directions with leader's prompting.	0 1 2 **3** 4 5	
	31. Are comfortable participating in activities in the presence of others.	0 1 2 **3** 4 5	
Associative	**Members**		4
	32. Begin to interact with some cooperation and competition.	0 1 2 3 **4** 5	
	33. Emphasize performance of activities over relationships.	0 1 2 3 **4** 5	
Basic Cooperative	**Members**		3
	34. Activity motivated by some self-interest.	0 1 2 **3** 4 5	
	35. Can identify and meet group goals with socially acceptable actions.	0 1 2 **3** 4 5	
Supportive Cooperative	**Members**		0
	36. Enjoy equality and compatibility between members.	**0** 1 2 3 4 5	
	37. Participate in mutual need satisfaction around expression of feelings similar to others.	**0** 1 2 3 4 5	
Mature	**Members**		0
	38. Maintain a balance between activity performance and interaction with group members.	**0** 1 2 3 4 5	
	39. Discuss serious topics (e.g., ethics, politics, health).	**0** 1 2 3 4 5	

Case Example 4.9. Psychiatric Inpatient-Unit Goal-Setting Group

Note. Many members in this group have a diagnosis of schizophrenia.

Setting: The setting is an occupational therapy inpatient-unit room with a table and chairs. Individualized goal ratings are on index cards.

Activities:

- Checking back on goal cards from previous week and evaluating activities or progress made on goals over the past week. Rating also commented on by two other group members.
- Discussion of each individual's goals by setting new goals for next week and short-term and long-term goals.

Interaction: Group members listen to each other's goals in cooperation with group aims. Most say they achieved their short-term goals for the week. Members are mostly pleased with themselves in terms of meeting goals. The group environment is pleasant as communication is exchanged. Some goals are set for postdischarge. Group members express the desire to leave the hospital, which the occupational therapist supports. Interaction is dry, without any creative initiative in roles played by members.

The group sets limits on one member whose goals are unrealistic (trying to achieve too much in dieting in a brief period of time). The group assists the member in setting a realistic goal. The participation in the group follows a structured format that produces a highly organized exchange. The group is very invested in the format for goal setting. Each person speaks briefly, and no one dominates the conversation. Group members defer to the occupational therapist in terms of her judgment on goals. The tone of the group is emotionally low key.

(See Social Profile Form for Case Example 4.9.)

Interpretation of Profile Ratings: Although the interactive exchange is structured in this group (by the goal cards), this group achieves solid associative and basic cooperative levels in which they express the goal to leave the hospital. Very little expression of emotion occurs, except for feelings about the inappropriate diet goal.

Case Example 4.9. Psychiatric Inpatient-Unit Goal-Setting Group

Topic 1: Activity participation: How do the activities influence group interactions?

0 = *Never*   1 = *Rarely*   2 = *Sometimes*   3 = *Frequently*   4 = *Almost always*   5 = *Always*

Level	Item Description	Score	Average
Parallel	**The activities provide**		
	1. Only little sharing of activity with group members.	0 1 2 3 4 5	3
	2. Only familiar activities that encourage performance of the activity, not group interaction.	0 1 2 3 4 5	
Associative	**The activities include**		
	3. Engagement in short-term activities.	0 1 2 3 4 5	4
	4. Joining in shareable activities with group members.	0 1 2 3 4 5	
	5. Enjoyment of activities between group members.	0 1 2 3 4 5	

(Continued)

Level	Item Description	Score	Average
Basic Cooperative	**The activities focus on**		3
	6. Longer, more complex activities.	0 1 2 **3** 4 5	
	7. The reflection of group goals and acceptable actions.	0 1 2 3 4 5	
	8. Completion of activities.	0 1 2 3 4 5	
	9. Opportunities to begin group problem solving.	0 1 2 3 4 5	
Supportive Cooperative	**The activities focus on**		0
	10. Attempts to satisfy others' emotional needs by words and actions.	**0** 1 2 3 4 5	
	11. Attempts to satisfy member's emotional needs by words and actions in addition to participation in the group activity.	**0** 1 2 3 4 5	
	12. Members select the activities.	**0** 1 2 3 4 5	
Mature	**The activities provide**		0
	13. Balance between emotional and performance needs of members.	**0** 1 2 3 4 5	
	14. Usually high-level performance, discussion, or product.	**0** 1 2 3 4 5	

Topic 2: Social interaction: How do group members interact with each other?

0 = *Never*   1 = *Rarely*   2 = *Sometimes*   3 = *Frequently*   4 = *Almost always*   5 = *Always*

Level	Item Description	Score	Average
Parallel	**Members interact**		2
	15. Very little with other people.	0 1 **2** 3 4 5	
	16. With minimal mutual stimulation or awareness.	0 1 **2** 3 4 5	
	17. With observance of parallel group rules.	0 1 **2** 3 4 5	
	18. Minimal verbal or nonverbal exchange between group members.	0 1 **2** 3 4 5	
Associative	**Members have been observed**		4
	19. Seeking activity assistance from others.	0 1 2 3 **4** 5	
	20. Giving concrete assistance willingly.	0 1 2 3 **4** 5	
	21. Understanding give and take in associative rules.	0 1 2 3 **4** 5	
Basic Cooperative	**Members interact by**		3
	22. Beginning to express ideas and meet needs of others.	0 1 2 **3** 4 5	
	23. Experimenting with group member roles (e.g., talker, initiator, listener).	0 1 2 **3** 4 5	
	24. Acting as though they have a right to be group members.	0 1 2 **3** 4 5	
	25. Respecting others' rights and basic cooperative rules.	0 1 2 **3** 4 5	
Supportive Cooperative	**Members have been observed to**		0
	26. Encourage self-expression of feelings in others.	**0** 1 2 3 4 5	
	27. Express positive and negative feelings.	**0** 1 2 3 4 5	
	28. Demonstrate caring about others in the group.	**0** 1 2 3 4 5	
Mature	**Members can**		0
	29. Assume a variety of member and leader roles without prompting.	**0** 1 2 3 4 5	

Topic 3: Group membership and roles: Do members feel they belong in the group?

0 = *Never*   1 = *Rarely*   2 = *Sometimes*   3 = *Frequently*   4 = *Almost always*   5 = *Always*

Level	Item Description	Score	Average
Parallel	**Members**		
	30. Appear to trust leaders and others; follow directions with leader's prompting.	0 1 2 **3** 4 5	3
	31. Are comfortable participating in activities in the presence of others.	0 1 2 **3** 4 5	
Associative	**Members**		
	32. Begin to interact with some cooperation and competition.	0 1 2 3 **4** 5	4
	33. Emphasize performance of activities over relationships.	0 1 2 3 **4** 5	
Basic Cooperative	**Members**		
	34. Activity motivated by some self-interest.	0 1 2 3 **4** 5	4
	35. Can identify and meet group goals with socially acceptable actions.	0 1 2 3 **4** 5	
Supportive Cooperative	**Members**		
	36. Enjoy equality and compatibility between members.	**0** 1 2 3 4 5	0
	37. Participate in mutual need satisfaction around expression of feelings similar to others.	**0** 1 2 3 4 5	
Mature	**Members**		
	38. Maintain a balance between activity performance and interaction with group members.	**0** 1 2 3 4 5	0
	39. Discuss serious topics (e.g., ethics, politics, health).	**0** 1 2 3 4 5	

Case Example 4.10. Psychiatric Inpatient Drug Abuse Prevention-of-Relapse Group

Setting: The setting is a psychiatric inpatient-unit group occupational therapy room. Handouts are available titled *Preventing Relapse.*

Activities: Members read the handout that describes relapse and list possible symptoms as warning signs of relapse. The handout includes a section in which the group members are to fill in four columns with headings "When I experience," "My response," "My change/plan," and "What my significant others can do to help." Discussion of what people are willing to share with the group takes place.

Interaction: Members try to follow instructions on the handout to describe relapse symptoms that arise. They indicate their usual response to the symptoms and their planned future efforts. Members speak to each other in respectful tones.

Some members are open about their repeated efforts to prevent relapse despite frequent past relapse. One member shares that he feels depressed. Members do not directly address this member's feelings of depression, but another person describes feelings of weakness before relapse. Most members can participate in the role of sharing feelings that are mentioned in the handout. It is not clear whether the group could express emotions on their own without the outline or the support of the occupational therapist.

Verbal discussion of goals follow the handout outline. Leadership is invested in the therapist, although some members are dominant in participating in the conversation. Members collaboratively set goals with input from other group members. Members seem pleased to be group members. No indication within the group exchange suggests that they are enabling each other to relapse.

(Continued)

Case Example 4.10. Psychiatric Inpatient Drug Abuse Prevention-of-Relapse Group

Topic 1: Activity participation: How do the activities influence group interactions?

0 = *Never*   1 = *Rarely*   2 = *Sometimes*   3 = *Frequently*   4 = *Almost always*   5 = *Always*

Level	Item Description	Score	Average
Parallel	**The activities provide** 1. Only little sharing of activity with group members. 2. Only familiar activities that encourage performance of the activity, not group interaction.	0 1 **2** 3 4 5 0 1 **2** 3 4 5	2
Associative	**The activities include** 3. Engagement in short-term activities. 4. Joining in shareable activities with group members. 5. Enjoyment of activities between group members.	0 1 2 **3** 4 5 0 1 2 **3** 4 5 0 1 2 **3** 4 5	3
Basic Cooperative	**The activities focus on** 6. Longer, more complex activities. 7. The reflection of group goals and acceptable actions. 8. Completion of activities. 9. Opportunities to begin group problem solving.	0 1 2 3 **4** 5 0 1 2 3 **4** 5 0 1 2 3 **4** 5 0 1 2 3 **4** 5	4
Supportive Cooperative	**The activities focus on** 10. Attempts to satisfy others' emotional needs by words and actions. 11. Attempts to satisfy member's emotional needs by words or actions in addition to participation in the group activity. 12. Members select the activities.	0 1 **2** 3 4 5 0 1 **2** 3 4 5 0 1 **2** 3 4 5	2
Mature	**The activities provide** 13. Balance between emotional and performance needs of members. 14. Usually high-level performance, discussion, or product.	**0** 1 2 3 4 5 **0** 1 2 3 4 5	0

Topic 2: Social interaction: How do group members interact with each other?

0 = *Never* 1 = *Rarely* 2 = *Sometimes* 3 = *Frequently* 4 = *Almost always* 5 = *Always*

Level	Item Description	Score	Average
Parallel	**Members interact**		2
	15. Very little with other people.	0 1 **2** 3 4 5	
	16. With minimal mutual stimulation or awareness.	0 1 **2** 3 4 5	
	17. With awareness of parallel group rules.	0 1 **2** 3 4 5	
	18. Minimal verbal or nonverbal exchange among group members.	0 1 **2** 3 4 5	
Associative	**Members have been observed**		4
	19. Seeking activity assistance from others.	0 1 2 3 **4** 5	
	20. Giving concrete assistance willingly.	0 1 2 3 **4** 5	
	21. Understanding give and take in associative rules.	0 1 2 3 **4** 5	
Basic Cooperative	**Members interact by**		3
	22. Beginning to express ideas and meet needs of others.	0 1 2 **3** 4 5	
	23. Experimenting with group member roles (e.g., talker, initiator, listener).	0 1 2 **3** 4 5	
	24. Acting as though they have a right to be group members.	0 1 2 **3** 4 5	
	25. Respecting others' rights and basic cooperative rules.	0 1 2 **3** 4 5	
Supportive Cooperative	**Members have been observed to**		2
	26. Encourage self-expression of feelings in others.	0 1 **2** 3 4 5	
	27. Express positive and negative feelings.	0 1 **2** 3 4 5	
	28. Demonstrate caring about others in the group.	0 1 **2** 3 4 5	
Mature	**Members can**		0
	29. Assume a variety of member and leader roles without prompting.	**0** 1 2 3 4 5	

Topic 3: Group membership and roles: Do members feel they belong in the group?

0 = *Never* 1 = *Rarely* 2 = *Sometimes* 3 = *Frequently* 4 = *Almost always* 5 = *Always*

Level	Item Description	Score	Average
Parallel	**Members**		2
	30. Appear to trust leaders and others; follow directions with leader's prompting.	0 1 **2** 3 4 5	
	31. Are comfortable participating in activities in the presence of others.	0 1 **2** 3 4 5	
Associative	**Members**		3
	32. Begin to interact with some cooperation and competition.	0 1 2 **3** 4 5	
	33. Emphasize performance of activities over relationships.	0 1 2 **3** 4 5	
Basic Cooperative	**Members**		4
	34. Activity motivated by some self-interest.	0 1 2 3 **4** 5	
	35. Can identify and meet group goals with socially acceptable actions.	0 1 2 3 **4** 5	
Supportive Cooperative	**Members**		2
	36. Enjoy equality and compatibility between members.	0 1 **2** 3 4 5	
	37. Participate in mutual need satisfaction around expression of feelings similar to others.	0 1 **2** 3 4 5	
Mature	**Members**		0
	38. Maintain a balance between activity performance and interaction with group members.	**0** 1 2 3 4 5	
	39. Discuss serious topics (e.g., ethics, politics, health).	**0** 1 2 3 4 5	

Case Example 4.11. Adolescent Basketball Game in School Courtyard

Setting: The setting is a high school courtyard, with six neighborhood boys. Two occupational therapy students co-led the group.

Activity: Spontaneous pick-up game, with three players on each team The usual teams of kids who know each other have been playing today for an hour.

Interaction: Boys call out to each other for plays and scores and several technical fouls. They call out strategies and negative and aggressive names to the opposite team. Players encourage their own team members and curse at their own mistakes. One team member hogs the ball at times instead of playing as a unit; others call him on it. They decide to take a time out.

Statements: "Here, over here." "Don't call what you are going to do." "Hey!" (on being bumped) "Five to three." "Get out of here." "Can't even shoot straight." "I'm off today." "What's wrong with you?" "Don't hog the ball." "Winners." "Let's take a time out." "Feed the ace." "Box out that big dude." "Don't let him penetrate."

(See Social Profile Form for Case Example 4.11.)

Interpretation of Profile Ratings: This group of 12- to 14-year-olds playing basketball in a school courtyard is organized by players engaging in longer basketball games for the day with a core of team members that has played over months and years. They enjoy the complex activity of the game's strategy and problem solve changes in a time-out. They select the activity and understand the give-and-take of team roles. For the most part, they respect each other's rights and follow the game rules. They experiment with roles in the group related to calling one player the "ace" and another player the "intruder." They demonstrate equality and recognize some feelings of other members, which is possible because they have known each other for an extended period. Their ratings range from the associative to the supportive cooperative levels.

Case Example 4.11. Adolescent Basketball Game in School Courtyard

Topic 1: Activity participation: How do the activities influence group interactions?

0 = *Never*   1 = *Rarely*   2 = *Sometimes*   3 = *Frequently*   4 = *Almost always*   5 = *Always*

Level	Item Description	Score	Average
Parallel	**The activities provide**		0
	1. Only little sharing of activity with group members.	0 1 2 3 4 5	
	2. Only familiar activities that encourage performance of the activity, not group interaction.	0 1 2 3 4 5	
Associative	**The activities include**		3
	3. Engagement in short-term activities.	0 1 2 3 4 5	
	4. Joining in shareable activities with group members.	0 1 2 3 4 5	
	5. Enjoyment of activities between group members.	0 1 2 3 4 5	
Basic Cooperative	**The activities focus on**		4
	6. Longer, more complex activities.	0 1 2 3 4 5	
	7. The reflection of group goals and acceptable actions.	0 1 2 3 4 5	
	8. Completion of activities.	0 1 2 3 4 5	
	9. Opportunities to begin group problem solving.	0 1 2 3 4 5	

(Continued)

Level	Item Description	Score	Average
Supportive Cooperative	**The activities focus on**		2
	10. Attempts to satisfy others' emotional needs by words and actions.	0 1 **2** 3 4 5	
	11. Attempts to satisfy member's emotional needs by words and actions in addition to participation in the group activity.	0 1 **2** 3 4 5	
	12. Members select the activities.	0 1 **2** 3 4 5	
Mature	**The activities provide**		0
	13. Balance between emotional and performance needs of members.	**0** 1 2 3 4 5	
	14. Usually high-level performance, discussion, or product.	**0** 1 2 3 4 5	

Topic 2: Social interaction: How do group members interact with each other?

0 = *Never*   1 = *Rarely*   2 = *Sometimes*   3 = *Frequently*   4 = *Almost always*   5 = *Always*

Level	Item Description	Score	Average
Parallel	**Members interact**		0
	15. Very little with other people.	**0** 1 2 3 4 5	
	16. With minimal mutual stimulation or awareness.	**0** 1 2 3 4 5	
	17. With observance of parallel group rules.	**0** 1 2 3 4 5	
	18. Minimal verbal or nonverbal exchange among group members.	**0** 1 2 3 4 5	
Associative	**Members have been observed**		4
	19. Seeking activity assistance from others.	0 1 2 3 **4** 5	
	20. Giving concrete assistance willingly.	0 1 2 3 **4** 5	
	21. Understanding give and take in associative rules.	0 1 2 3 **4** 5	
Basic Cooperative	**Members interact by**		4
	22. Beginning to express ideas and meet needs of others.	0 1 2 3 **4** 5	
	23. Experimenting with group member roles (e.g., talker, initiator, listener).	0 1 2 3 **4** 5	
	24. Acting as though they have a right to be group members.	0 1 2 3 **4** 5	
	25. Respecting others' rights and basic cooperative rules.	0 1 2 3 **4** 5	
Supportive Cooperative	**Members have been observed to**		3
	26. Encourage self-expression of feelings in others.	0 1 2 **3** 4 5	
	27. Express positive and negative feelings.	0 1 2 **3** 4 5	
	28. Demonstrate caring about others in the group.	0 1 2 **3** 4 5	
Mature	**Members can**		0
	29. Assume a variety of member and leader roles without prompting.	**0** 1 2 3 4 5	

Topic 3: Group membership and roles: Do members feel they belong in the group?

0 = *Never* 1 = *Rarely* 2 = *Sometimes* 3 = *Frequently* 4 = *Almost always* 5 = *Always*

Level	Item Description	Score	Average
Parallel	**Members** 30. Appear to trust leaders and others; follow directions with leader's prompting.	**0** 1 2 3 4 5	0
	31. Are comfortable participating in activities in the presence of others.	**0** 1 2 3 4 5	
Associative	**Members** 32. Begin to interact with some cooperation and competition.	0 1 **2** 3 4 5	2
	33. Emphasize performance of activities over relationships.	0 1 **2** 3 4 5	
Basic Cooperative	**Members** 34. Activity motivated by some self-interest.	0 1 2 3 **4** 5	4
	35. Can identify and meet group goals with socially acceptable actions.	0 1 2 3 **4** 5	
Supportive Cooperative	**Members** 36. Enjoy equality and compatibility between members.	0 1 2 3 **4** 5	4
	37. Participate in mutual need satisfaction around expression of feelings similar to others.	0 1 2 3 **4** 5	
Mature	**Members** 38. Maintain a balance between activity performance and interaction with group members.	**0** 1 2 3 4 5	0
	39. Discuss serious topics (e.g., ethics, politics, health).	**0** 1 2 3 4 5	

Case Example 4.12. Adult Psychiatric Problem-Solving Group

Setting: The setting is a unit ward activity room, with group members sitting around a large table. There are 11 clients.

Activities: The group decides on an interactive problem-solving activity that may have a cultural, ethical, or political focus. The group selects an ethical dilemma regarding the decision of whether to terminate an unwanted pregnancy. The group discusses options, ethics, and social implications for a boyfriend.

Interaction: Group members comment on options of abortion versus adoption. They discuss the health of the mother and how much of this decision is up to the father. They express shock that the mother died of an illegal, botched abortion. Group members seem to care about the outcome and process of decision making.

Statements: "It's her body. She can make the decision." "What about the father?" "I keep changing my mind about the situation." "Was she in good health?" "The mother's death was just an accident." "It's not easy to decide." "Taking responsibility for her life and the baby's life is complicated." "How many weeks or months old was the fetus?" "Should we call it a *fetus* or *baby*?" "She was trapped in this pregnancy." "Each person can make his or her own choices."

(See Social Profile Form for Case Example 4.12.)

Interpretation of Profile Ratings: This group makes the effort to discuss a serious topic and balance activity performance with interaction with group members, but it does so at a moderate level of social participation interaction. Those in the group assume various member and leadership roles without prompting. The group's focus is on joint problem solving and listening to each other while maintaining their own perspective. Their spectrum of interaction spans four levels of participation, including some mature-level comments of concern for others' welfare and the ability to see several sides of a dilemma.

Case Example 4.12. Adult Psychiatric Problem-Solving Group

Topic 1: Activity participation: How do the activities influence group interactions?

0 = *Never*   1 = *Rarely*   2 = *Sometimes*   3 = *Frequently*   4 = *Almost always*   5 = *Always*

Level	Item Description	Score	Average
Parallel	**The activities provide**		0
	1. Only little sharing of activity with group members.	**0** 1 2 3 4 5	
	2. Only familiar activities that encourage performance of the activity, not group interaction.	**0** 1 2 3 4 5	
Associative	**The activities include**		1
	3. Engagement in short-term activities.	0 **1** 2 3 4 5	
	4. Joining in shareable activities with group members.	0 **1** 2 3 4 5	
	5. Enjoyment of activities between group members.	0 **1** 2 3 4 5	
Basic Cooperative	**The activities focus on**		4
	6. Longer, more complex activities.	0 1 2 3 **4** 5	
	7. The reflection of group goals and acceptable actions.	0 1 2 3 **4** 5	
	8. Completion of activities.	0 1 2 3 **4** 5	
	9. Opportunities to begin group problem solving.	0 1 2 3 **4** 5	
Supportive Cooperative	**The activities focus on**		3
	10. Attempts to satisfy others' emotional needs by words or actions.	0 1 2 **3** 4 5	
	11. Attempts to satisfy member's emotional needs by words or actions in addition to participation in the group activity.	0 1 2 **3** 4 5	
	12. Members select the activities.	0 1 2 **3** 4 5	
Mature	**The activities provide**		2
	13. Balance between emotional and performance needs of members.	0 1 **2** 3 4 5	
	14. Usually high-level performance, discussion, or product.	0 1 **2** 3 4 5	

Topic 2: Social interaction: How do group members interact with each other?

0 = *Never*   1 = *Rarely*   2 = *Sometimes*   3 = *Frequently*   4 = *Almost always*   5 = *Always*

Level	Item Description	Score	Average
Parallel	**Members interact**		0
	15. Very little with other people.	**0** 1 2 3 4 5	
	16. With minimal mutual stimulation or awareness.	**0** 1 2 3 4 5	
	17. With observance of parallel group rules.	**0** 1 2 3 4 5	
	18. Minimal verbal or nonverbal exchange between group members.	**0** 1 2 3 4 5	
Associative	**Members have been observed**		2
	19. Seeking activity assistance from others.	0 1 **2** 3 4 5	
	20. Giving concrete assistance willingly.	0 1 **2** 3 4 5	
	21. Understanding give and take in associative rules.	0 1 **2** 3 4 5	
Basic Cooperative	**Members interact by**		3
	22. Beginning to express ideas and meet needs of others.	0 1 2 **3** 4 5	
	23. Experimenting with group member roles (e.g., talker, initiator, listener).	0 1 2 **3** 4 5	
	24. Acting as though they have a right to be group members.	0 1 2 **3** 4 5	
	25. Respecting others' rights and basic cooperative rules.	0 1 2 **3** 4 5	

(Continued)

Level	Item Description	Score	Average
Supportive Cooperative	**Members have been observed to** 26. Encourage self-expression of feelings in others. 27. Express positive and negative feelings. 28. Demonstrate caring about others in the group.	0 1 2 3 4 5 0 1 2 3 4 5 0 1 2 3 4 5	3
Mature	**Members can** 29. Assume a variety of member and leader roles without prompting.	0 1 2 3 4 5	2

Topic 3: Group membership and roles: Do members feel they belong in the group?

0 = *Never*   1 = *Rarely*   2 = *Sometimes*   3 = *Frequently*   4 = *Almost always*   5 = *Always*

Level	Item Description	Score	Average
Parallel	**Members** 30. Appear to trust leaders and others; follow directions with leader's prompting. 31. Are comfortable participating in activities in the presence of others.	0 1 2 3 4 5 0 1 2 3 4 5	0
Associative	**Members** 32. Begin to interact with some cooperation and competition. 33. Emphasize performance of activities over relationships.	0 1 2 3 4 5 0 1 2 3 4 5	0
Basic Cooperative	**Members** 34. Activity motivated by some self-interest. 35. Can identify and meet group goals with socially acceptable actions.	0 1 2 3 4 5 0 1 2 3 4 5	2
Supportive Cooperative	**Members** 36. Enjoy equality and compatibility between members. 37. Participate in mutual need satisfaction around expression feelings similar to others.	0 1 2 3 4 5 0 1 2 3 4 5	3
Mature	**Members** 38. Maintain a balance between activity performance and interaction with group members. 39. Discuss serious topics (e.g., ethics, politics, health).	0 1 2 3 4 5 0 1 2 3 4 5	3

Case Example 4.13. High School Dance Decorating Committee Group

Setting: The High School Dance Decorating Committee is decorating the gym for the Valentine's Day Dance. The area has construction, crepe paper, and poster paper; balloons; and plastic heart shapes. Music is on in background.

Activities: Students discuss what decorations to use and what to put where. They make an elaborate heart entrance around the main door, with flowers for all to wear and name tags. They put up streamers, balloons, hearts, cupids, arrows, and images of hands holding hands. They play their favorite music. They create subcommittees to do various aspects of the gym areas.

Interaction: Almost all committee members participate and seem to know each other well after many years in school together. Subcommittees work well together, although they may represent small cliques. One subcommittee borrows tape and Blu-Tack® from another subcommittee in a congenial manner. Someone offered to get more supplies from the office and the pharmacy.

(Continued)

Case Example 4.13. High School Dance Decorating Committee Group *(cont.)*

Each subcommittee respects the other's designs and decorations. The Dance Decorating Committee chair asks each subcommittee how it wants to decorate their area or portion of the gym. One subcommittee teases the door heart design subcommittee in a lighthearted way. Lots of banter occurs as the groups work and play at shaping their designs. The participants say they like this type of open dance without specific, paired dates.

The pace of the group's work is leisurely, because the exchange of conversation is perceived by some students as just as important as how the finished gym looks. The group probably takes more than an hour longer to complete the task than is necessary, but they seem to be enjoying each other's company. They finally finish decorating about 2 hours before the dance.

(See Social Profile for Case Example 4.13.)

Interpretation of Profile Ratings: Members of the Dance Decorating Committee care about their joint event and each other. They place their relationships above the achievement of the gym decor. They express feelings to each other about their ideas and emotions. Sometimes they balance the activity performance and interaction with group members, but overall they prefer a supportive cooperative mode of working. Their ratings span four levels of participation, from some associative to mature levels of interaction. However, because the task is less important than their camaraderie, the mature-level rating is lower than the supportive cooperative–level rating in some areas.

Case Example 4.13. High School Dance Decorating Committee Group

Topic 1: Activity participation: How do the activities influence group interactions?

0 = Never   *1 = Rarely*   *2 = Sometimes*   *3 = Frequently*   *4 = Almost always*   *5 = Always*

Level	Item Description	Score	Average
Parallel	**The activities provide**		0
	1. Only little sharing of activity with group members.	0 1 2 3 4 5	
	2. Only familiar activities that encourage performance of the activity, not group interaction.	0 1 2 3 4 5	
Associative	**The activities include**		2
	3. Engagement in short-term activities.	0 1 2 3 4 5	
	4. Joining in shareable activities with group members.	0 1 2 3 4 5	
	5. Enjoyment of activities between group members.	0 1 2 3 4 5	
Basic Cooperative	**The activities focus on**		4
	6. Longer, more complex activities.	0 1 2 3 4 5	
	7. The reflection of group goals and acceptable actions.	0 1 2 3 4 5	
	8. Completion of activities.	0 1 2 3 4 5	
	9. Opportunities to begin group problem solving.	0 1 2 3 4 5	
Supportive Cooperative	**The activities focus on**		4
	10. Attempts to satisfy others' emotional needs by words or actions.	0 1 2 3 4 5	
	11. Attempts to satisfy member's emotional needs by words or actions in addition to participation in the group activity.	0 1 2 3 4 5	
	12. Members select the activities.	0 1 2 3 4 5	
Mature	**The activities provide**		2
	13. Balance between emotional and performance needs of members.	0 1 2 3 4 5	
	14. Usually high-level performance, discussion, or product.	0 1 2 3 4 5	

Topic 2: Social interaction: How do group members interact with each other?

| 0 = Never | 1 = Rarely | 2 = Sometimes | 3 = Frequently | 4 = Almost always | 5 = Always |

Level	Item Description	Score	Average
Parallel	**Members interact**		0
	15. Very little with other people.	**0** 1 2 3 4 5	
	16. With minimal mutual stimulation or awareness.	**0** 1 2 3 4 5	
	17. With observation of parallel group rules.	**0** 1 2 3 4 5	
	18. Minimal verbal or nonverbal exchange among group members.	**0** 1 2 3 4 5	
Associative	**Members have been observed**		3
	19. Seeking activity assistance from others.	0 1 2 **3** 4 5	
	20. Giving concrete assistance willingly.	0 1 2 **3** 4 5	
	21. Understanding give and take in associative rules.	0 1 2 **3** 4 5	
Basic Cooperative	**Members interact by**		4
	22. Beginning to express ideas and meet needs of others.	0 1 2 3 **4** 5	
	23. Experimenting with group member roles (e.g., talker, initiator, listener).	0 1 2 3 **4** 5	
	24. Acting as though they have a right to be group members.	0 1 2 3 **4** 5	
	25. Respecting others' rights and basic cooperative rules.	0 1 2 3 **4** 5	
Supportive Cooperative	**Members have been observed to**		4
	26. Encourage self-expression of feelings in others.	0 1 2 3 **4** 5	
	27. Express positive and negative feelings.	0 1 2 3 **4** 5	
	28. Demonstrate caring about others in the group.	0 1 2 3 **4** 5	
Mature	**Members can**		4
	29. Assume a variety of member and leader roles without prompting.	0 1 2 3 **4** 5	

Topic 3: Group membership and roles: Do members feel they belong in the group?

| 0 = Never | 1 = Rarely | 2 = Sometimes | 3 = Frequently | 4 = Almost always | 5 = Always |

Level	Item Description	Score	Average
Parallel	**Members**		0
	30. Appear to trust leaders and others; follow directions with leader's prompting.	**0** 1 2 3 4 5	
	31. Are comfortable participating in activities in the presence of others.	**0** 1 2 3 4 5	
Associative	**Members**		1
	32. Begin to interact with some cooperation and competition.	0 **1** 2 3 4 5	
	33. Emphasize performance of activities over relationships.	0 **1** 2 3 4 5	
Basic Cooperative	**Members**		4
	34. Activity motivated by some self-interest.	0 1 2 3 **4** 5	
	35. Can identify and meet group goals with socially acceptable actions.	0 1 2 3 **4** 5	
Supportive Cooperative	**Members**		4
	36. Enjoy equality and compatibility between members.	0 1 2 3 **4** 5	
	37. Participate in mutual need satisfaction around expression of feelings similar to others.	0 1 2 3 **4** 5	
Mature	**Members**		2
	38. Maintain a balance between activity performance and interaction with group members.	0 1 **2** 3 4 5	
	39. Discuss serious topics (e.g. ethics, politics, health).	0 1 **2** 3 4 5	

Case Example 4.14. Community Senior Reminiscence Group

Setting: The setting is a large room in a senior center located in a city. Chairs are around a large table. The group consists of 12 well older adult members. The group is a community activity group.

Activities: Participants are discussing memories of 50 years ago.

Interaction: The occupational therapist describes the perspective that toward the end of life, people often look for meaning in their lives across their life span. The therapist asks the individuals to close their eyes and go back 50 years or more in time. Members are asked to describe a significant event at that period of their lives.

Several individuals or couples talk about dating and their wedding day, describing them as happy times. They state that they worked hard. Others speak about the birth of their children as their most memorable reminiscence, pleased that they established a family. Several talk about holiday gatherings and the significance of having all their relatives around them. Discussion sounds enjoyable. Members commented on others' memories in a sympathetic manner.

One couple remains silent and is asked by the therapist and the group about their experiences 50 years ago. They stated they do not want to darken the happy environment of the group by telling about their experiences in Europe during the 1940s. The group encourages them to share their history, stating they are there to listen to others' life experiences, even if they were painful.

The couple speak of imprisonment and the loss of relatives; emotions caused by these events are expressed. Other group members are supportive in their responses. Group members ask appropriate questions and talk about their regrets for the events and losses that occurred in the lives of the couple, who express appreciation for the heartfelt emotions shared by the group. They say they have not talked about this grief outside their family. The therapist asks whether they feel they need further support or follow-up. They say they will let the therapist know next week.

Interpretation of Profile Ratings: This group is considerate of others' feelings, can discuss serious topics, and can balance task completion and interaction with group members. They are far beyond just beginning to cooperate and can give abstract, nonconcrete assistance to each other. For that reason, the group has some ratings in the basic cooperative level that are lower than their ratings at the supportive cooperative and mature levels of participation.

(See the Social Profile form for Case Example 4.14.)

Case Example 4.14. Community Senior Reminiscence Group

Topic 1: Activity participation: How do the activities influence group interactions?

0 = *Never*   1 = *Rarely*   2 = *Sometimes*   3 = *Frequently*   4 = *Almost always*   5 = *Always*

Level	Item Description	Score	Average
Parallel	**The activities provide**		
	1. Only little sharing of activity with group members.	0 1 2 3 4 5	0
	2. Only familiar activities that encourage performance of the activity, not group interaction.	0 1 2 3 4 5	
Associative	**The activities include**		
	3. Engagement in short-term activities.	0 1 2 3 4 5	3
	4. Joining in shareable activities with group members.	0 1 2 3 4 5	
	5. Enjoyment of activities between group members.	0 1 2 3 4 5	

(Continued)

Level	Item Description	Score	Average
Basic Cooperative	**The activities focus on** 6. Longer, more complex activities. 7. The reflection of group goals and acceptable actions. 8. Completion of activities. 9. Opportunities to begin group problem solving.	0 1 2 3 4 5 0 1 2 3 4 5 0 1 2 3 4 5 0 1 2 3 4 5	4
Supportive Cooperative	**The activities focus on** 10. Attempts to satisfy others' emotional needs by words and actions. 11. Attempts to satisfy member's emotional needs by words and actions in addition to participation in the group activity. 12. Members select the activities.	0 1 2 3 4 5 0 1 2 3 4 5 0 1 2 3 4 5	4
Mature	**The activities provide** 13. Balance between emotional and performance needs of members. 14. Usually high-level performance, discussion, or product.	0 1 2 3 4 5 0 1 2 3 4 5	4

Topic 2: Social interaction: How do group members interact with each other?

0 = Never   *1 = Rarely*   *2 = Sometimes*   *3 = Frequently*   *4 = Almost always*   *5 = Always*

Level	Item Description	Score	Average
Parallel	**Members interact** 15. Very little with other people. 16. With minimal mutual stimulation or awareness. 17. With observance of parallel group rules. 18. Minimal verbal or nonverbal exchange among group members.	**0** 1 2 3 4 5 **0** 1 2 3 4 5 **0** 1 2 3 4 5 **0** 1 2 3 4 5	0
Associative	**Members have been observed** 19. Seeking activity assistance from others. 20. Giving concrete assistance willingly. 21. Understanding give and take in associative rules.	0 1 2 3 4 5 0 1 2 3 4 5 0 1 2 3 4 5	3
Basic Cooperative	**Members interact by** 22. Beginning to express ideas and meet needs of others. 23. Experimenting with group member roles (e.g., talker, initiator, listener). 24. Acting as though they have a right to be group members. 25. Respecting others' rights and basic cooperative rules.	0 1 2 3 4 5 0 1 2 3 4 5 0 1 2 3 4 5 0 1 2 3 4 5	4
Supportive Cooperative	**Members have been observed to** 26. Encourage self-expression of feelings in others. 27. Express positive and negative feelings. 28. Demonstrate caring about others in the group.	0 1 2 3 4 5 0 1 2 3 4 5 0 1 2 3 4 5	4
Mature	**Members can** 29. Assume a variety of member and leader roles without prompting.	0 1 2 3 4 5	4

Topic 3: Group membership and roles: Do members feel they belong in the group?

0 = Never   1 = Rarely   2 = Sometimes   3 = Frequently   4 = Almost always   5 = Always

Level	Item Description	Score	Average
Parallel	**Members** 30. Appear to trust leaders and others; follow directions with leader's prompting.	0 1 2 3 4 5	0
	31. Are comfortable participating in activities in the presence of others.	0 1 2 3 4 5	
Associative	**Members** 32. Begin to interact with some cooperation and competition.	0 1 2 3 4 5	0
	33. Emphasize performance of activities over relationships.	0 1 2 3 4 5	
Basic Cooperative	**Members** 34. Activity motivated by some self-interest.	0 1 2 3 4 5	3
	35. Can identify and meet group goals with socially acceptable actions.	0 1 2 3 4 5	
Supportive Cooperative	**Members** 36. Enjoy equality and compatibility between members.	0 1 2 3 4 5	4
	37. Participate in mutual need satisfaction around expression of feelings similar to others.	0 1 2 3 4 5 0 1 2 3 4 5	
Mature	**Members** 38. Maintain a balance between activity performance and interaction with group members.	0 1 2 3 4 5	4
	39. Discuss serious topics (e.g., ethics, politics, health).	0 1 2 3 4 5	

Preparation for Group Observations for New Group Leaders

In clinical student fieldwork training, it has been found that students and some beginning occupational therapists need to learn group observation skills to assess social participation (Donohue, 2001). One method that has proven successful has been to practice observations of groups for 30-minute periods, examining seven major aspects or factors of group participation:

1. *Cooperation* is the attitude and willingness to assist others in their efforts and to work together with the leader, the other members, and activities and materials of the day. Despite differences of opinion, members can agree to disagree to continue with their joint activities.

2. *Norms* are the rules, values, customs, standards, or guidelines of the group within the cultural expectations of gender, race, religion, nationality, and age. They are neutral in value.

3. *Group roles* are the positions or functions assumed or acquired by people through effort during the process of being a group member.

For example, Bales's (1950) roles of initiator, information or opinion seeker or giver, co-ordinator, orienter, evaluator, energizer, procedural technician, encourager, harmonizer, gatekeeper, expediter, standard setter, follower, aggressor, blocker, recognition seeker, self-confessor, playboy, dominator, help seeker, and special interest pleader are some roles exhibited in groups.

4. *Communication* consists of giving or exchanging information or messages with others in verbal and nonverbal ways. It can be formal and structured or informal and emotional.

5. *Activities behaviors* are the actions performed in carrying out tasks, goals, or activities: the doing, the motion, the pace, and the degree of investment or involvement in the activity.

6. *Power and leadership* in a group is the manifestation of the ability to act and do activities or to speak with authority in a group to direct or influence steps taken jointly.

7. *Motivation and attraction* in a group is the desire to find the people, activities, time,

and location of the group appealing (Bales, 1950; Cartwright & Zander, 1968; Cole, 2012; Johnson & Johnson, 2009; Schwartzberg et al., 2008; Yalom & Leszcz, 2005).

Goals set by individuals and by the group jointly can be observed and inquired about by the observer. Exhibit 4.1 is an observation sheet that potential evaluators can use to improve their observation skills.

Note that the social behaviors being observed may correctly belong under more than one factor. Abstract and complex psychosocial factors may overlap, and observers may accurately record a single behavior under more than one factor. If questions arise, observers should confer with a supervisor or experienced group leader for clarification.

The following examples show how evaluators can practice their observation skills by using the observation sheet in Exhibit 4.1. These examples are based on three case examples previously presented in this chapter (Case Examples 4.7, 4.9, and 4.10).

Case Example 4.7. Adult Psychiatric Inpatient Grooming Group

Eight patients at lowest level of function with many acute symptoms and dressed in pajamas or green gowns, and 3 dressed in day clothes; 11 group members, 2 students, 1 aide, 1 therapist.

- **Cooperation:** Six men began to shave (3 were at sink with mirror), others used mirrors on table with basins; all eventually were involved; no conflicts occurred in using materials; they took turns; enough materials for all: razors, mirrors, basins (student took care of watching and collecting razors).
- **Norms:** Radio was on; 1 woman at table had a woolen hat on and showed humor; therapist knows everyone's names; a couple of patients knew one to two names.
- **Roles:** Initially, only 1 woman was present; she expressed the emotion that she felt alone; therapist called another woman from the unit to make the lone woman feel more comfortable; solitary shaver by window talked to self, smiling to self as he stood by the radio after shaving.

- **Communication:** Radio was on; woman laughed, showed humor ("Do I have to share?"). She said she wants a job; said she had her own business, talked a lot; second woman has humor, too; 4 people at the table talked in pairs (2 men and 2 women); some talked to the therapist; 1 woman spoke to the whole group; the nature of the group does not lend itself to formal discussion at the end.
- **Activity behaviors:** One member changed the radio station, and no one said anything; group used mirrors on wall, table, plastic pans, razors, lotion, shaving cream; some stood talking, listening to the radio, and not finishing shaving, and many left cream on their face and clothes until told by students or therapist. Other patients may have noticed but did not comment on shaving cream on the face; women did nail activity with nail polish.
- **Power and leadership:** One person changed the radio station. The therapist asked if anyone could remember more than 2 names of others in group. Therapist asked, "Did you clean up your work area?" Power invested in the therapist.
- **Motivation and attraction:** Therapist knows names of all members. Therapist said, "Say 5 names aloud for a prize." One man who appeared unmotivated was standing with just shaving cream on his face; later shaved after face was prepared. Group did not comment on results of grooming, whether it made them attractive or was an attractive activity.

Social participation analysis

- **Parallel:** Most of the activity of the group was at this level, because few group members talked to each other. They were shaving next to each other and did not ask for feedback from others regarding how they looked or how they were doing; women doing nails were less parallel in action because they were talking more to each other. *60 percent at this level? (Note.* Use SP for more exact rating.)
- **Associative:** There was some socialization by men hanging out near the radio who exchanged a few words. Men took turns with sharing shaving

materials without conflict. A few patients knew 1 or 2 names of others in the group but did not tell others about shaving cream on the face. *25% at this level?* (*Note.* Use SP for more exact rating.)

- **Basic cooperative:** Some discussion among women whose task of doing nails required less concentration than shaving. Two men at the table shaving talked together. One woman laughed and showed humor. One woman spoke to the whole group without receiving a response. No one knew 5 names of group members. *15% at this level?* (*Note.* Use SP for more exact rating.)
- **Supportive cooperative:** (Little evidence of emotion expressed except for laughter and one nonsupportive statement of humor, "Do I have to share?")
- **Mature:** (No evidence of this level of interaction.)

Case Example 4.9. Psychiatric Inpatient-Unit Goal-Setting Group

- **Cooperation:** Members took turns stating goals; they listened to others and reality-tested unrealistic goals (e.g., eating 10 fruits per day); some goals they saw as out of their control, for example, taking medication, roommate selection, and having to check in with nurses on the unit every 20 minutes, which was annoying, but they did it to be cooperative.
- **Norms:** Members took turns speaking; they understood norm of short-term goals and expectation to set goals of a reasonable nature; they did not always understand what was reasonable in terms of realistic goals.
- **Roles:** To evaluate others' goals: All chimed in regarding having 10 fruits per day; there were parallel roles in goal-setting statements and in answering the therapist's question, "What did you get out of this group?" by way of speaking only to the therapist and not to each other.
- **Communication:** There were some comments among members across the group; most communication was directed toward therapist; group laughed when 1 person mentioned a goal of eating 10 fruits in 1 day.

- **Activity behaviors:** The members were alert to activity of goal selection but not always appropriate in actual selection of goals; needed guidance in judging frequency and scope of issues under their control.
- **Power and leadership:** Members tried to influence 1 person with unreasonable, concrete goal regarding eating 10 fruits per day; members did not do as well in influencing others in some instances despite the group's version of the goal itself being reasonable (e.g., medication, nurses, roommates).
- **Motivation and attraction:** Members wanted to get better and wanted to leave the hospital; they perceived the achievement of these goals as a way to attain discharge; they wanted to interact with people across the group because they found participation attractive.

Social participation analysis

- **Parallel:** Attention focused on leader for the most part and on other members; therefore, social participation is beyond the parallel level in this group.
- **Associative:** Brief interactions occurred with the group leader. Members took turns speaking. There were some interactions with other group members. *25% of behaviors at this level?*
- **Basic cooperative:** The members understood the norms of the group: to have and state short-term goals for hospitalization. Members appeared to want to get better. They laughed at a member who wanted to eat fruit as a goal; they eventually helped the member with this unrealistic goal in a basic, concrete manner. Members needed prompting to respond to general goals of the group meeting, such as what the members achieved in the group. Most members focused on reasonable goals regarding medication, nurses, and roommate relationships, but it was not easy to convince other group members of the need for practical goals. *60% of behaviors at this level?*
- **Supportive cooperative:** Some wanted to communicate with members across the group. They did express thoughts about unrealistic goals: All members chimed in. *Brief behaviors at this level? 15%?*

- **Mature:** (No evidence of mature-level group participation in this session.)

Case Example 4.10. Psychiatric Inpatient Drug Abuse Prevention-of-Relapse Group

- **Cooperation:** Members tried to follow the columns on the handout "Preventing Relapse" to describe symptoms, their usual response to symptoms, and future efforts planned. Some degree of helping each other occurred through discussion. One person added to the discussion that he or she was isolated before a recent relapse.
- **Norms:** Most interactions were with the group leader. Some group members were open about repeated efforts not to relapse. Members had a respectful tone in their responses to shared information. One member was able to share well enough to admit having had depression.
- **Roles:** Most members entered the role of sharing feelings by following the outline. One-half of the group was more verbal than the other half, who did not speak were but attentive. The group was all male. Did that affect the group? One person expressed feelings of weakness before relapse.
- **Communication:** Most communication was directed toward the group leader. The group drew from a possible list of symptoms on the handout for discussion. Would the group be able to express emotions on their own or without the therapist or handout? Why is this question important?
- **Activity behaviors:** Verbal discussion of goals followed outline on the handout, which was used to direct the discussion of possible symptoms or warnings of relapse. The group shared feelings following the columns on the outline in an orderly manner without much creative discussion.
- **Power and leadership:** Directing the group seems central to the therapist. Several members were somewhat dominant in the conversation. It is unclear whether they could conduct or coordinate the group on their own without a therapist or professional leader if given guidelines.
- **Motivation and attraction:** Members wanted to set goals collaboratively with input from other

group members. Members seemed pleased to be group members and valued others' opinions and camaraderie. No indication of enabling each other to relapse was revealed in this group. Is this being hidden during hospitalization?

Social participation analysis

- **Parallel:** (Discussion and interaction was at this level for some members.)
- **Associative:** (Discussion consisted merely of words or phrases at this level.) Half the group appears to function at this level because they do not speak to each other. Most of the group interaction is directed toward the therapist. *30% of behaviors at this level?*
- **Basic cooperative:** Members have a respectful tone toward each other. Most members use the outline to guide their discussion interaction and appear dependent on the handout to identify symptoms. Discussion of goals and of possible symptoms warning of relapse is concretely processed by using the handout guidelines. Several members play dominant roles in the conversation. This group is probably not ready to conduct the group by joint leadership with so many quiet members and with 2 very assertive members. *55% of behaviors at this level?*
- **Supportive cooperative:** Desire to set goals collaboratively with input from others in the group illustrates some performance at this level. Admissions of depression and symptoms in the past, discussion of efforts to prevent relapse, and feelings of weakness before relapse also represent some performance at this level. No appearance of overt symptoms of jokes or sarcasm or "enabling" each other to relapse into drug use. *15% of behaviors at this level?*
- **Mature:** (No evidence of mature interaction whereby the group actively helps each other and takes turns in assistance roles.)

Summary

This chapter provided guidelines and examples for the interpretation of 14 group cases at a variety of levels and in a variety of settings. These cases illustrate the

SP's flexibility in assessing levels of participation as being at parallel, associative, basic cooperative, supportive cooperative, and mature levels of interaction. Readers and researchers are invited to expand the use of the SP within their activity group practice settings.

A section for students and new therapists includes an observation sheet as a guide to developing skills as a broad-based accurate rater by searching for behaviors providing evidence of cooperation, norms, group roles, communication, activity behaviors, power and leadership, motivation for the activity, attraction to the group, and identification of group and individual goals while observing groups for a half-hour.

Feedback on and research using the SP is encouraged. The author can be contacted at MaryVDonohue@gmail.com. Further information is available at: www.Social-Profile.com.

References

American Educational Research Association, American Psychological Association, & National Council on Measurement in Education. (1992). *Standards for educational and psychological testing* (3rd ed.). Washington, DC: Author.

Aureli, T., & Colecchia, N. (1996). Day care experience and free play behavior in preschool children. *Journal of Applied Developmental Psychology, 17,* 1–10. http://dx.doi.org/10.1016/S0193-3973(96)90002-7

Bales, R. (1950). *Interaction process analysis.* Reading, MA: Addison-Wesley.

Bandura, A. (1973). *Aggression: A social learning analysis.* Englewood Cliffs, NJ: Prentice-Hall.

Bandura, A. (1977). *Social learning theory.* New York: General Learning Press.

Bandura, A. (1986). *Social foundations of thought and action: A social cognitive theory.* Englewood Cliffs, NJ: Prentice-Hall.

Bar-On, R., Maree, J. G., & Elias, M. J. (Eds.). (2007). *Educating people to be emotionally intelligent.* Westport, CT: Praeger.

Bellack, A. S., Mueser, K. T., Gingerich, S., & Agresta, J. (1997). *Social skills training for schizophrenia: A step-by-step guide.* New York: Guilford Press.

Bernard, H. R. (2000). *Social research methods: Qualitative and quantitative approaches.* Newbury Park, CA: Sage.

Borg, B., & Bruce, M. A. (1991). *The group system: The therapeutic activity group in occupational therapy.* Thorofare, NJ: Slack.

Bredenkamp, S., & Copple, C., (Eds.). (2009). *Developmentally appropriate practice in early childhood programs, serving children from birth through age eight.* Washington, DC: National Association for the Education of Young Children.

Brooks, D. (2011). *The social animal: The hidden sources of love, character and achievement.* New York: Random House.

Brown, J. A. C. (1971). *Freud and the post-Freudians.* London: Penguin.

Bruce, M. A., & Borg, B. (2002). *Psychosocial occupational therapy: Frames of reference for intervention* (3rd ed.). Thorofare, NJ: Slack.

Buchner, A., Erdfelder, E., & Faul, F. (1997). *How to use G*Power.* Retrieved from www.psycho.uni-duesseldorf.de/aap/projects/gpower/how_to_use_gpower.html

Burns, N., & Grove, S. K. (2009). *The practice of nursing research: Conduct, critique, and utilization.* Philadelphia: W. B. Saunders.

Carmines, E. G., & Zeller, R. A. (1991). *Reliability and validity assessment.* Newbury Park, CA: Sage.

Cartwright, D., & Zander, A. (Eds.). (1968). *Group dynamics: Research and theory* (3rd ed.). New York: Harper & Row.

Case-Smith, J., & Archer, L. (2008, January 21). School-based services for students with emotional disturbance. Findings and recommendations. *OT Practice,* pp. 17–21.

Centers for Disease Control and Prevention. (2008). *Social capital.* Retrieved from www.cdc.gov/healthyplaces/healthtopics/social.htm

Christiakis, N. A., & Fowler, J. H. (2011). *Connected.* New York: Little Brown.

Cohen, J. (Ed.). (2004). *Caring classrooms/intelligent schools: The social emotional education of young children.* New York: Teachers College Press.

Cohen, J. (2006). Social, emotional, ethical, and academic education: Creating a climate for learning participation in democracy and well-being. *Harvard Educational Review, 76,* 201–237.

Cohen, R. J., Swerdlik, M. E., & Phillips, S. M. (1995). *Psychological testing and assessment: An introduction to tests and measurements* (3rd ed.). Mountain View, CA: Mayfield.

Cole, M. B. (2012). *Group dynamics in occupational therapy: The theoretical basis and practice application of group treatment.* Thorofare, NJ: Slack.

Cole, M. B., & Donohue, M. V. (2011). *Social participation in occupational contexts: In schools, clinics, and communities.* Thorofare, NJ: Slack.

Coleman, J. S. (1988). Social capital in the creation of human capital. *American Journal of Sociology, 94*(Suppl.), S95–S120. http://dx.doi.org/10.1086/228943

Corey, M. S., & Corey, G. (1997). *Groups: Process and practice* (5th ed.). New York: Brooks/Cole.

Crick, N. R., & Dodge, K. A. (1994). A review and reformulation of social-information processing mechanisms in children's social adjustment. *Psychological Bulletin, 115,* 74–101. http://dx.doi.org/10.1037/0033-2909.115.1.74

Deci, E. L., & Ryan, R. M. (2000). The what and why of goal pursuits: Human needs and self-determination of behavior. *Psychological Inquiry, 11,* 227–268. http://dx.doi.org/10.1207/S15327965PLI1104_01

Devine, J., Cohen, J., & Elias, M. J. (2007). *Making your school safe: Strategies to protect children and promote learning.* New York: Teachers College Press.

Dildine, G. C. (1972). Characteristics of a mature group. In U. Delworth, E. H. Rudow, & J. Taub (Eds.), *Crisis center/hotline: A guidebook to beginning and operating* (pp. 79–81). Springfield, IL: Charles C Thomas.

Donohue, M. V. (1999). Theoretical bases of Mosey's group interactions skills. *Occupational Therapy International, 6,* 35–51. http://dx.doi.org/10.1002/oti.87

Donohue, M. V. (2001). Group co-leadership by occupational therapy students in community centers: Learning transitional roles. *Occupational Therapy in Health Care, 15,* 85–98. http://dx.doi.org/10.1300/J003v15n01_09

Donohue, M. V. (2003). Group profile studies with children: Validity measures and item analysis. *Occupational Therapy in Mental Health, 19,* 1–23. http://dx.doi.org/10.1300/J004v19n01_01

Donohue, M. V. (2005). Social Profile: Assessment of validity and reliability with preschool children. *Canadian Journal of Occupational Therapy, 72,* 164–175.

Donohue, M. V. (2006). Interrater reliability of the Social Profile: Assessment of community and psychiatric group participation. *Australian Occupational Therapy Journal, 54,* 49–58. doi: 10.1111/j.1440-1630.2006.00622.x

Donohue, M. V. (2010a). Evaluation of social participation. In K. Sladyk, K. Jacobs, & N. MacRae (Eds.), *Occupational therapy essentials for clinical competence* (pp. 151–162). Thorofare, NJ: Slack.

Donohue, M. V. (2010b). *Test–retest reliability of the Social Profile.* Unpublished manuscript.

Donohue, M. V., Hanif, H., & Wu Berns, L. (2011). An exploratory Study of Social Participation in Occupational Therapy Groups. *Mental Health Special Interest Section Quarterly, 34*(3), 1–4.

Duncombe, L. W., & Howe, M. C. (1995). Group treatment: Goals, tasks, and economic implications. *American Journal of Occupational Therapy, 49,* 199–205. http://dx.doi.org/10.5014/ajot.49.3.199

Dusseldorf University. (2010). *Means: Difference between two dependent means (matched pairs).* Dusseldorf, Germany: Heinrich Heine Universität Düsseldorf, Institut for Experimentelle Psychologie. Retrieved from www.psycho.uni-duesseldorf.de/abteilungen/aap/gpower3/user-guide-by-distribution/t/means_difference_between_two_dependent

Erikson, E. H. (1968). *Identity: Youth and crisis.* New York: Norton.

Fantuzzo, J., Sutton-Smith, B., Atkins, M., Meyers, R., Stevenson, H., Coolahan, K., et al. (1996). Community-based resilient peer treatment of withdrawn maltreated preschool children. *Journal of Consulting and Clinical Psychology, 64,* 1377–1386. http://dx.doi.org/10.1037/0022-006X.64.6.1377

Field, T. (1984). Play behaviors of handicapped children who have friends. In T. Field, J. L. Roopnarine, & M. Segal (Eds.), *Friendship in normal and handicapped children* (pp. 153–162). Norwood, NJ: Ablex.

Fukuyama, F. (1995). *Trust: The social virtues and the creation of prosperity.* New York: Free Press.

Fukuyama, F. (1999, November). *Social capital and civil society.* Paper presented at the IMF Conference on Second Generation Reforms, Washington, DC. Retrieved from www.imf.org/external/pubs/ft/seminar/1999/reforms/fukuyama.htm

Garnier, C., & Latour, A. (1994). Analysis of group process: Cooperation of preschool children. *Canadian Journal of Behavioural Science/Revue Canadienne des Sciences, 26,* 365–384. http://dx.doi.org/10.1037/0008-400X.26.3.365

Gbowee, L., & Mithers, C. (2011). *Mighty be our powers. How sisterhood, prayer, and sex changed a nation at war.* New York: Beast Books.

Geselle, A. (1940). *The first five years of life: A guide to the study of the preschool child.* New York: Harper.

Gliner, J. A., & Morgan, G. A. (2000). *Research methods in applied settings. An integrated approach to design and analysis.* Mahwah, NJ: Erlbaum.

Gough, H. G. (1987). *California Psychological Inventory: Administrator's guide* (3rd ed.). Palo Alto, CA: Consulting Psychologists Press.

Guralnick, M. J., & Groom, J. M. (1987). The peer relations of mildly delayed and nonhandicapped preschool children in mainstreamed playgroups. *Child Development, 58,* 1556–1572. http://dx.doi.org/10.2307/1130695

Guralnick, M. J., & Groom, J. M. (1988). Friendships of preschool children in mainstreamed playgroups. *Developmental Psychology, 24,* 595–604. http://dx.doi.org/10.1037/0012-1649.24.4.595

Hanifan, L. J. (1916). The Rural School Community Center. *Annals of the American Academy of Political and Social Science, 67,* 130–138.

Henninger, M. L. (1994). Planning for outdoor play. *Young Children, 4,* 10–15.

Hertz-Lazarowitz, R., Feitelson, D., Zahavi, S., & Hartup, W. W. (1981). Social interaction and social organization of Israeli five- to seven-year-olds. *International Journal of Behavioral Development, 4,* 143–155.

Howes, C. (1988). Peer interaction of young children. *Monographs of the Society for Research in Child Development, 53,* 1–88.

Hughes, F. P. (2009). *Children, play, and development* (4th ed.). Thousand Oaks, CA: Sage.

Illinois State Board of Education. (2008). *Illinois learning standard: Social/emotional learning (SEL).* Retrieved from www.isbe.net/ils/social_emotional/standards.htm

Jackson, J., Carlson, M., Mandel, D., Zemke, R., & Clark, F. (1998). Occupation in lifestyle redesign: The Well Elderly Study Occupational Therapy Program. *American Journal of Occupational Therapy, 52,* 326–336. http://dx.doi.org/10.5014/ajot.52.5.326

Jackson, L. L., & Arbesman, M. (2005). *Occupational therapy practice guidelines for children with behavioral and psychosocial needs.* Bethesda, MD: AOTA Press.

Jetten, J., Haslam, C., & Haslam, A. (Eds.). (2012). *The social cure: Identity, health, and well-being.* New York: Psychology Press.

Johnson, D. W., & Johnson, F. P. (2009). *Joining together: Group theory and group skills.* Boston: Allyn & Bacon.

Kam, C. M., Greenberg, M. T., & Kusche, C. A. (2004). Sustained effects of the PATHS curriculum on the social and psychological adjustment of children in special education. *Journal of Emotional and Behavioral Disorders, 12,* 66–78. http://dx.doi.org/10.1177/10634266040120020101

Kanas, N. (1966). *Group therapy for schizophrenic patients.* Washington, DC: American Psychiatric Press.

Kim, J., Kim, S. Y., & Kaslak, M. A. (2005). Teachers' understanding and uses of developmentally appropriate practice for young children in Korea. *Journal of Research in Childhood Education, 20,* 49–56. http://dx.doi.org/10.1080/02568540509594550

Kim, J. O., & Mueller, C. W. (1978). *Introduction to factor analysis: What it is and how to do it.* Newbury Park, CA: Sage.

Krantz, M. (1982). Sociometric awareness, social participation, and perceived popularity in preschool children. *Child Development, 53,* 376–379. http://dx.doi.org/10.2307/1128979

Lave, J. (1988). *Cognition in practice: Mind, mathematics and culture in everyday life.* Cambridge, England: Cambridge University Press.

Lifton, W. M. (1966). *Working with groups: Group process and individual growth.* New York: Wiley.

Lissitz, R. W., & Samuelsen, K. (2007). A suggested change in terminology and emphasis regarding validity and education. *Educational Researcher, 36,* 437–448. http://dx.doi.org/10.3102/0013189X07311286

MEERA: My Environmental Education Evaluation Resource Assistant. (2007). *Plan an evaluation.* Retrieved from http://meera.snre.umich.edu/plan-an-evaluation

Mezrich, B. (2010). *The accidental billionaires: The founding of Facebook.* New York: Anchor.

Miller, L. J. (Ed.). (1989). *Developing norm-referenced standardized tests.* New York: Haworth.

Miller, L. A., McIntire, S. A., & Lovler, R. L. (2011). *Foundations of psychological testing: A practical approach* (3rd ed.). Thousand Oaks, CA: Sage.

Miller, N., & Dollard, J. (1940). *Social learning and imitation.* New Haven, CT: Yale University Press.

Mosey, A. C. (1968). Recapitulation of ontogenesis: A theory for practice of occupational therapy. *American Journal of Occupational Therapy, 22,* 426–438.

Mosey, A. C. (1986). *Psychosocial components of occupational therapy.* New York: Raven Press.

Nachmias, D., & Nachmias, C. (2008). *Research methods in the social sciences.* New York: St. Martin's Press.

Neufeld, P. S. (2004, August 9). Enabling participation through community and population approaches. *OT Practice,* pp. CE1–CE8.

O'Neil, H., & Perez, R. (Eds.). (2007). *Computer games and team and individual learning.* Los Angeles: Elsevier Science.

Parten, M. B. (1932). Social participation among pre-school children. *Journal of Abnormal and Social Psychology, 27,* 243–269. doi: 10.1037/h0074524

Passi, L. E. (1998). *A guide to creative group programming in the psychiatric day hospital.* Binghamton, NY: Haworth Press.

Petrakos, H., & Howe, N. (1996). The influence of the physical design of the dramatic play center on children's play. *Early Childhood Research Quarterly, 11,* 63–77. http://dx.doi.org/10.1016/S0885-2006(96)90029-0

Piaget, J. (1956). *Les stades du developpment intellectuel de l'enfant et de l'adolescent* [The stages of intellectual development of the child and adolescent]. In *Le probleme des stades en psychologie de l'enfant: Troisieme symposium de l'association psychologique scientifique de langue francaise, Genève 1955* (pp. 33–42). Paris: Presses Universitaires de France.

Polit, D. F., & Hungler, B. P. (1995). *Nursing research: Principles and methods.* Philadelphia: Lippincott.

Portes, A. (1998). Social capital. Its origins and application in modern sociology. *Annual Review of Sociology, 24,* 1–24. http://dx.doi.org/10.1146/annurev.soc.24.1.1

Posthuma, B. W. (2002). *Small groups in counseling and therapy: Process and leadership* (4th ed.). Needham Heights, MA: Allyn & Bacon.

Precin, P. (1999). *Living skills recovery workbook.* Boston: Butterworth Heinemann.

Rao, N., Moely, B. E., & Lockman, J. J. (1987). Increasing social participation in preschool social isolates. *Journal of Clinical Child Psychology, 16,* 178–183. http://dx.doi.org/10.1207/s15374424jccp1603_1

Raphael-Greenfield, E., Shteyler, A., Silva, M. R., Canine, P. G., Soo, S., Rotonda, E. C., & Patrone, D. O. (2011). Hardwired for groups: Students and clients in the classroom and clinic. *Mental Health Special Interest Quarterly, 34,* 1–4.

Remocker, A. J., & Sherwood, E. T. (1999). *Action speaks louder: A handbook of structured group techniques* (6th ed.). New York: Churchill Livingston.

Robinson, C. C., Anderson, G. T., Porter, C. L., Hart, C. H., & Wouden-Miller, M. (2003). Sequential patterns in the natural play of preschool children: Is parallel play a bridge to other play states? *Early Childhood Research Quarterly, 18,* 3–21. http://dx.doi.org/10.1016/S0885-2006(03)00003-6

Salo-Chydenius, S. (1996). Changing helplessness to coping: An exploratory study of social skills training with individuals with long-term mental illness. *Occupational Therapy International, 3,* 174–189. http://dx.doi.org/10.1002/oti.35

Santrock, J. W. (2007). *A topical approach to life-span development* (3rd ed.). New York: McGraw-Hill.

Saracho, O. N. (1993). A factor analysis of young children's play. *Early Child Development and Care, 84,* 91–102. http://dx.doi.org/10.1080/0300443930840108

Schwartzberg, S. L. (2002). *Interactive reasoning in the practice of occupational therapy.* Upper Saddle River, NJ: Prentice Hall.

Schwartzberg, S. L., Howe, M. C., & Barnes, M. A. (2008). *Groups: Applying the functional group model.* Philadelphia: F. A. Davis.

Schwartzberg, S. L., Howe, M., & McDermott, A. (1982). A comparison of three treatment group formats for facilitating social interaction. *Occupational Therapy in Mental Health, 2,* 1–16.

Shrout, P. E., & Fleiss, J. L. (1979). Intraclass correlations: Uses in assessing rater reliability. *Psychological Bulletin, 86,* 420–428. http://dx.doi.org/10.1037/0033-2909.86.2.420

Spector, P. E. (1992). *Summated rating scale construction: An introduction.* Newbury Park, CA: Sage.

SPSS. (2008). *Version 17.* Chicago: SPSS, Inc.

Stein, F., Rice, M. S., & Cutler, S. K. (2013). *Clinical research in occupational therapy* (5th ed.). Clifton Park, NY: Delmar.

Tanta, K. J., Deitz, J. C., White, O., & Billingsley, F. (2005). The effects of peer-play level on initiations and responses of preschool children with delayed play skills. *American Journal of Occupational Therapy, 59,* 437–445. http://dx.doi.org/10.5014/ajot.59.4.437

Vygotsky, L. S. (1978). *Mind in society.* Cambridge, MA: Harvard University Press.

Weinberg, S., & Goldberg, K. (1990). *Statistics for the behavioral sciences.* New York: Cambridge University Press.

World Bank. (2008). *Social capital.* Retrieved from http://Web.worldbank.org/Wbsite/external/topics/extsocial development

World Health Organization. (2001). *International classification of functioning, disability and health (ICF).* Geneva: Author.

World Health Organization. (2007). *International classification of functioning, disability and health—Children and youth version (ICF–CY).* Geneva: Author.

Yaffee, R. A. (1998). *Enhancement of reliability analysis: Application of intraclass correlations with SPSS/ Windows v. 8.* New York: New York University.

Yalom, I. D., & Leszcz, M. (2005). *The theory and practice of group psychotherapy* (3rd ed.). New York: Basic Books.

Zins, J. E., & Elias, M. J. (2007). A commentary on social emotional learning: Promoting the development of all students. *Journal of Educational and Psychological Consultation, 17,* 257–262. http://dx.doi .org/10.1080/10474410701346758

APPENDIX A   Social Profile: Children's Version

Assessment of Activity Participation, Social Interaction, and Membership Roles in a Group

Purpose: The Social Profile (SP) was created to assess group-level functioning during activities. Data from the SP organize a group's developmental and functional levels with a standard numerical coding system.

Three Levels of Group Participation

Parallel. Group members play, move, or work side by side but *do not interact* with each other.
Associative. Group members approach each other *briefly* in verbal and nonverbal interactions during play, activity, or work.
Basic cooperative. Group members jointly select, implement, and execute *longer* play, activity, or work tasks for reasons of *mutual self-interest* in the goal, project, or fellow members.

Scoring Instructions

1. **Select a group session to observe and record the observations on the SP.**
   - Choose an activity group session typical for this group that is at an average level of participation for the group or for an individual being observed in the group. Observe the group or individual for at least a half-hour.
   - Or, after observing at least 3 sessions of a group, mentally average its level of participa-

tion in your mind, and record it numerically on one SP form.
   - Rate the group's or individual's behavioral levels of participation that occur at the parallel, associative, or basic cooperative levels. Rate those levels that pertain to the group or individual across all the relevant levels of the SP for that group or individual
   - On the pages titled "Activity Participation," "Social Interaction," and "Group Membership," using the Likert scale, rate items as the following:
     - 0 = *Never*
     - 1 = *Rarely*
     - 2 = *Sometimes*
     - 3 = *Frequently*
     - 4 = *Almost always*
     - 5 = *Always.*
   - *Note.* Reading and rating the items at the parallel level requires additional information, because it is a pregroup assembly of noninteractive people. Parallel-level items are designed to describe a setting in which people are present in a space together and engaged in a solitary activity next to other people without conversation. The items reflect participants' limited awareness of others present by using words such as *only, very little,* and *minimal verbal exchange or awareness of others* and describe individuals who are dependent on the leader and yet comfortable in the presence of others. The term *parallel* for this profile describes parallel activities without any conversation.
   - When individuals or groups socially participate at associative or basic cooperative levels, they should receive a 0 at the parallel level to indicate that they are not at the parallel level.

Note. Three levels of social participation adapted from "Social Participation Among Pre-School Children," by M. B. Parten, 1932, *Journal of Abnormal and Social Psychology, 27,* pp. 243–269. Copyright © 1932, by the American Psychological Association. Adapted with permission.

(This absence of social participation at this level has been validated by research described in the SP manual.)

2. **Carry the average of the ratings to the top of the Summary Sheet.**

3. **Copy ratings from the top of the Summary Sheet, and create a graph on the page following it.** The ratings may be horizontally or vertically connected as line graphs. This final step is optional.

Name of Group: _____

Topic 1. Activity participation: How do the activities influence the children's group interactions?

0 = *Never*   1 = *Rarely*   2 = *Sometimes*   3 = *Frequently*   4 = *Almost always*   5 = *Always*

Level	Item Description	Score	Average
Parallel	**The activities provide**		
	1. Only little sharing of activity with group members.	0 1 2 3 4 5	
	2. Only familiar activities that encourage performance of the activity, not group interaction.	0 1 2 3 4 5	
Associative	**The activities include**		
	3. Engagement in short-term activities.	0 1 2 3 4 5	
	4. Joining in shareable activities with group members.	0 1 2 3 4 5	
	5. Enjoyment of activities between group members.	0 1 2 3 4 5	
Basic Cooperative	**The activities focus on**		
	6. Longer, more complex activities.	0 1 2 3 4 5	
	7. The reflection of group goals and acceptable actions.	0 1 2 3 4 5	
	8. Completion of activities.	0 1 2 3 4 5	
	9. Opportunities to begin group problem solving.	0 1 2 3 4 5	

Topic 2. Social interaction: How do the children in the group interact with each other?

0 = *Never*   1 = *Rarely*   2 = *Sometimes*   3 = *Frequently*   4 = *Almost always*   5 = *Always*

Level	Item Description	Score	Average
Parallel	**Members interact**		
	10. Very little with other children.	0 1 2 3 4 5	
	11. With minimal mutual stimulation or awareness.	0 1 2 3 4 5	
	12. With awareness of group membership rules.	0 1 2 3 4 5	
	13. Minimal verbal or nonverbal exchange among group members.	0 1 2 3 4 5	
Associative	**Members have been observed**		
	14. Seeking activity assistance from others.	0 1 2 3 4 5	
	15. Giving concrete assistance willingly.	0 1 2 3 4 5	
	16. Understanding give and take in associative rules.	0 1 2 3 4 5	
Basic Cooperative	**Members interact by**		
	17. Beginning to express ideas and meet needs of others.	0 1 2 3 4 5	
	18. Experimenting with group member roles (e.g., talker, initiator, listener).	0 1 2 3 4 5	
	19. Acting as though they have a right to be group members.	0 1 2 3 4 5	
	20. Respecting others' rights and basic cooperative rules.	0 1 2 3 4 5	

Topic 3. Group membership and roles: Do the children feel they belong in the group?

0 = Never   1 = Rarely   2 = Sometimes   3 = Frequently   4 = Almost always   5 = Always

Level	Item Description	Score	Average
Parallel	**Members** 21. Appear to trust leaders and others; follow directions with leader's prompting.	0 1 2 3 4 5	
	22. Are comfortable participating in activities in the presence of others.	0 1 2 3 4 5	
Associative	**Members** 23. Begin to interact with some cooperation and competition.	0 1 2 3 4 5	
	24. Emphasize performance of activities over relationships.	0 1 2 3 4 5	
Basic Cooperative	**Members in the group** 25. Activity motivated by some self-interest.	0 1 2 3 4 5	
	26. Can identify and meet group goals with socially acceptable actions.	0 1 2 3 4 5	

Social Profile Summary Sheet

Individual or group name: _____
Social activity: _____

Directions: Transfer the average scores for each level from each of the three topics of the SP to the appropriate box below. In the summary column, average each level's average score. You may average the summaries if the result appears to be clinically or educationally meaningful. On the next page, graph the results of the Likert scores within each level to obtain a profile of the group's social participation during activity interaction. The graph step is optional.

Level	Topic 1. Activity Participation	Topic 2. Social Interaction	Topic 3. Group Membership	Summary Average of Topics 1, 2, and 3
Basic Cooperative				
Associative				
Parallel				

If meaningful, average of summaries: _____

Average summary scores can be interpreted in the following way:
- **5** = *mature level of social or group participation*
- **4–5** = *supportive cooperative to mature levels of social or group participation*
- **3–4** = *basic cooperative to supportive cooperative levels of social or group participation*
- **2–3** = *associative to basic cooperative levels of social or group participation*
- **1–2** = *parallel to associative levels of social or group participation*
- **1** = *parallel level of social group participation.*

Composite Graph: Activity Participation, Social Interaction, and Group Membership

Directions: Plot the numbers from the summary sheet on the graph below, and connect points in a line graph. You may plot the graph horizontally or vertically.

Level		Activity Participation	Social Interaction	Group Membership
Basic Cooperative	5			
	4			
	3			
	2			
	1			
	0			
Associative	5			
	4			
	3			
	2			
	1			
	0			
Parallel	5			
	4			
	3			
	2			
	1			
	0			

APPENDIX B Social Profile: Adult/Adolescent Version

Assessment of Activity Participation, Social Interaction, and Membership Roles in a Group

Purpose: The Social Profile (SP) was created to assess group-level functioning during activities. This version can be self-administered by individual group members or by an outside evaluator. Data from the SP organize a group's developmental and functional levels with a standard numerical coding system.

Five Levels of Social Participation

Parallel. Group members play, move, or work side by side but *do not interact* with each other.

Associative. Group members approach each other *briefly* in verbal and nonverbal interactions during play, activity, or work.

Basic cooperative. Group members jointly select, implement, and execute *longer* play, activity, or work tasks for reasons of *mutual self-interest* in the goal, project, or fellow members.

Supportive cooperative. Group members are homogeneous and aim to fulfill their needs for mutual *emotional* satisfaction with the goals of play, activity, or work viewed as secondary. *Feelings* are frequently expressed.

Mature. The members of the group *take turns* in a variety of complementary *roles* to achieve the goals of the activity harmoniously and efficiently. The group combines basic cooperative and supportive cooperative interaction.

Note. The five levels of social participation are adapted from "Recapitulation of Ontogenesis: A Theory for Practice of Occupational Therapy," by A. C. Mosey, 1968, *American Journal of Occupational Therapy, 22,* pp. 426–438. Copyright © 1968, by the American Occupational Therapy Association. Adapted with permission. Also from "Social Participation Among Pre-School Children," by M. B. Parten, 1932, *Journal of Abnormal and Social Psychology, 27,* pp. 243–269. Copyright © 1932, by the American Psychological Association. Adapted with permission.

Scoring Instructions

1. **Select a group session to observe and record the observations on the SP.**
   - Choose an activity group session typical for this group that is at an average level of participation for the group or for an individual being observed in the group. Observe the group or individual for at least a half-hour.
   - Or, after observing at least 3 sessions of a group, mentally average its level of participation in your mind, and record it numerically on one SP form.
   - Rate the group's or individual's behavioral levels of participation that occur at the parallel, associative, basic cooperative, supportive cooperative, or mature levels. Rate those levels that pertain to the group or individual across all the relevant levels of the SP for that group or individual.
   - On the pages titled "Activity Participation," "Social Interaction," and "Group Membership," using the Likert scale, rate items as the following:
     - *0 = Never*
     - *1 = Rarely*
     - *2 = Sometimes*
     - *3 = Frequently*
     - *4 = Almost always*
     - *5 = Always.*

   - *Note.* Reading and rating the items at the parallel level requires additional information, because it is a pregroup assembly of noninteractive people. Parallel-level items are designed to describe a setting in which people are present in a space together and engaged in a solitary activity next to other people without conversation. The items reflect participants' limited awareness of others present by using words such as *only, very little,* and *minimal verbal exchange or awareness of others* and describe individuals who are dependent on the leader and yet comfortable in the presence of others. The term *parallel* for this profile describes parallel activities without any conversation.

- When individuals or groups socially participate at associative to mature levels, they can receive a 0 at the parallel level to indicate that they are not at the parallel level. (This absence of social

participation at this level has been validated by research described in the SP manual.) With higher-level groups, it is recommended to first rate the SP from the mature to supportive cooperative to basic cooperative levels and then consider the associative and parallel levels.

2. **Carry the average of the ratings to the top of the Summary Sheet.**
3. **Copy ratings from the top of the Summary Sheet, and create a graph on the page following it.** The ratings may be horizontally or vertically connected as line graphs. This final step is optional.

Name of Group: _____

Topic 1. Activity participation: How do the activities influence group interactions?

0 = *Never*   1 = *Rarely*   2 = *Sometimes*   3 = *Frequently*   4 = *Almost always*   5 = *Always*

Level	Item Description	Score	Average
Parallel	The activities provide		
	1. Only little sharing of activity with group members.	0 1 2 3 4 5	
	2. Only familiar activities that encourage performance of the activity, not group interaction.	0 1 2 3 4 5	
Associative	The activities include		
	3. Engagement in short-term activities.	0 1 2 3 4 5	
	4. Joining in shareable activities with group members.	0 1 2 3 4 5	
	5. Enjoyment of activities between group members.	0 1 2 3 4 5	
Basic Cooperative	The activities focus on		
	6. Longer, more complex activities.	0 1 2 3 4 5	
	7. The reflection of group goals and acceptable actions.	0 1 2 3 4 5	
	8. Completion of activities.	0 1 2 3 4 5	
	9. Opportunities to begin group problem solving.	0 1 2 3 4 5	
Supportive Cooperative	The activities focus on		
	10. Attempts to satisfy others' emotional needs by words or actions.	0 1 2 3 4 5	
	11. Attempts to satisfy member's emotional needs by words or actions in addition to participation in the group activity.	0 1 2 3 4 5	
	12. Members select the activities.		
Mature	The activities provide		
	13. Balance between emotional and performance needs of members.	0 1 2 3 4 5	
	14. Usually high-level performance, discussion, or product.	0 1 2 3 4 5	

Topic 2. Social interaction: How do group members interact with each other?

0 = *Never*   1 = *Rarely*   2 = *Sometimes*   3 = *Frequently*   4 = *Almost always*   5 = *Always*

Level	Item Description	Score	Average
Parallel	**Members interact**		
	15. Very little with other people.	0 1 2 3 4 5	
	16. With minimal mutual stimulation or awareness.	0 1 2 3 4 5	
	17. With observance of parallel group rules.	0 1 2 3 4 5	
	18. Minimal verbal or nonverbal exchange among group members.	0 1 2 3 4 5	
Associative	**Members have been observed**		
	19. Seeking activity assistance from others.	0 1 2 3 4 5	
	20. Giving concrete assistance willingly.	0 1 2 3 4 5	
	21. Understanding give and take in associative rules.	0 1 2 3 4 5	
Basic Cooperative	**Members interact by**		
	22. Beginning to express ideas and meet needs of others.	0 1 2 3 4 5	
	23. Experimenting with group member roles (e.g., talker, initiator, listener).	0 1 2 3 4 5	
	24. Acting as though they have a right to be group members.	0 1 2 3 4 5	
	25. Respecting others' rights and basic cooperative rules.	0 1 2 3 4 5	
Supportive Cooperative	**Members have been observed to**		
	26. Encourage self-expression of feelings in others.	0 1 2 3 4 5	
	27. Express positive and negative feelings.	0 1 2 3 4 5	
	28. Demonstrate caring about others in the group.	0 1 2 3 4 5	
Mature	**Members can**		
	29. Assume a variety of member and leader roles without prompting.	0 1 2 3 4 5	

Topic 3. Group membership and roles: Do members feel they belong in the group?

0 = *Never*   1 = *Rarely*   2 = *Sometimes*   3 = *Frequently*   4 = *Almost always*   5 = *Always*

Level	Item Description	Score	Average
Parallel	**Members**		
	30. Appear to trust leaders and others and follow directions with leader's prompting.	0 1 2 3 4 5	
	31. Are comfortable participating in activities in the presence of others.	0 1 2 3 4 5	
Associative	**Members**		
	32. Begin to interact with some cooperation and competition.	0 1 2 3 4 5	
	33. Emphasize performance of activities over relationships.	0 1 2 3 4 5	
Basic Cooperative	**Members**		
	34. Activity motivated by some self-interest.	0 1 2 3 4 5	
	35. Can identify and meet group goals with socially acceptable actions.	0 1 2 3 4 5	
Supportive Cooperative	**Members**		
	36. Enjoy equality and compatibility between members.	0 1 2 3 4 5	
	37. Participates in mutual need satisfaction around expression of feelings similar to others.	0 1 2 3 4 5	
Mature	**Members**		
	38. Maintain a balance between activity performance and interaction with group members.	0 1 2 3 4 5	
	39. Discuss serious topics (e.g., ethics, politics, health).	0 1 2 3 4 5	

Social Profile Summary Sheet

Individual or Group Name: _____

Social Activity: _____

Directions: Transfer the average scores for each level from each of the three topics of the SP to the appropriate box below. In the summary column, determine each level's average score. You may average the summaries if the result appears to be clinically or educationally meaningful. On the next page, graph the results of the Likert scores within each level to obtain a profile of the group's social participation during activity interaction. The graph step is optional.

Level	Topic 1. Activity Participation	Topic 2. Social Interaction	Topic 3. Group Membership	Summary Average of Topics 1, 2, 3
Mature				
Supportive Cooperative				
Basic Cooperative				
Associative				
Parallel				

If meaningful, average of summaries: _____

Average summary scores can be interpreted in the following way:
- **5** = *mature level of social or group participation*
- **4–5** = *supportive cooperative to mature levels of social or group participation*
- **3–4** = *basic cooperative to supportive cooperative levels of social or group participation*
- **2–3** = *associative to basic cooperative levels of social or group participation*
- **1–2** = *parallel to associative levels of social or group participation*
- **1** = *parallel level of social group participation.*

Composite Graph: Activity Participation, Social Interaction, and Group Membership

Directions: Plot the numbers from the summary sheet on the graph below, and connect points in a line graph. You may plot the graph horizontally or vertically.

Level		Activity Participation	Social Interaction	Group Membership
Mature	5			
	4			
	3			
	2			
	1			
	0			
Supportive Cooperative	5			
	4			
	3			
	2			
	1			
	0			
Basic Cooperative	5			
	4			
	3			
	2			
	1			
	0			
Associative	5			
	4			
	3			
	2			
	1			
	0			
Parallel	5			
	4			
	3			
	2			
	1			
	0			

Recommended Resources

The following resources provide guidance for goal setting and group social intervention after a group or individual in a group is rated using the Social Profile.

Web Resources

American Educational Research Association (AERA; www.aera.net): AERA has a Special Interest Group on social–emotional learning.

Collaborative for Academic, Social, and Emotional Learning (www.casel.org)

National School Climate Center (www.csee.net)

Reggio Emilia Program (www.lifeinitaly.com/potpourri/children-education.asp)

Social Profile Web site (www.Social-Profile.com)

Books and Articles

American Educational Research Association, American Psychological Association, & National Council on Measurement in Education. (1992). *Standards for educational and psychological testing* (3rd ed.). Washington, DC: Author.

American Occupational Therapy Association. (2004). Psychosocial aspects of occupational therapy (2004). *American Journal of Occupational Therapy, 58,* 660–672. http://dx.doi.org/10.5014/ajot.58.6.669

American Occupational Therapy Association. (2008). Occupational therapy practice framework: Domain and process (2nd ed.). *American Journal of Occupational Therapy, 62,* 625–683. http://dx.doi.org/105014/ajot.62.6.625

American Psychiatric Association. (2000). *The diagnostic and statistical manual of mental disorders* (4th ed., text rev.). Washington, DC: Author.

Bar-On, R., Maree, J. G., & Elias, M. J. (Eds.). (2007). *Educating people to be emotionally intelligent.* Westport, CT: Praeger.

Benight, C. C., & Bandura, A. (2004). Social cognitive theory of posttraumatic recovery: The role of perceived self-efficacy. *Behavior Research and Therapy, 42,* 1129–1148. http://dx.doi.org/10.1016/j.brat.2003.08.008

Black, D. R., Foster, E. S., & Tindall, J. A. (2011). *Evaluation of peer and prevention programs: A blueprint for successful design and implementation.* Clifton, NJ: Routledge.

Blum, R. W., McNeely, C. A., & Rinehart, P. M. (2002). *Improving the odds: The untapped power of schools to improve the health of teens.* Minneapolis: University of Minnesota, Center for Adolescent Health and Development.

Borg, B., & Bruce, M. A. (1991). *The group system: The therapeutic activity group in occupational therapy.* Thorofare, NJ: Slack.

Bredenkamp, S., & Copple, C. (Eds.). (2009). *Developmentally appropriate practice in early childhood programs, serving children from birth through age eight.* Washington, DC: National Association for the Education of Young Children.

Brown, C., & Stoffel, V. (Eds.). (2011). *Occupational therapy in mental health: A vision for participation.* Philadelphia: F. A. Davis.

Bruce, M. A., & Borg, B. (2002). *Psychosocial occupational therapy: Frames of reference for intervention* (3rd ed.). Thorofare, NJ: Slack.

Case-Smith, J., & Archer, L. (2008, January 21). School-based services for students with emotional disturbance. Findings and recommendations. *OT Practice,* pp. 17–21.

Christiakis, N. A., & Fowler, J. H. (2011). *Connected.* New York: Little Brown.

Cohen, J. (Ed.). (2004). *Caring classrooms/intelligent schools: The social emotional education of young children.* New York: Teachers College Press.

Cohen, J. (2006). Social, emotional, ethical, and academic education: Creating a climate for learning participation in democracy and well-being. *Harvard Educational Review, 76,* 201–237.

Cole, M. B. (2012). *Group dynamics in occupational therapy: The theoretical basis and practice application of group treatment.* Thorofare, NJ: Slack.

Cole, M. B., & Donohue, M. V. (2010). *Social participation in occupational contexts: In schools, clinics and communities.* Thorofare, NJ: Slack.

Corey, M. S., & Corey, G. (1997). *Groups: Process and practice* (5th ed.). New York: Brooks/Cole.

Crick, N. R., & Dodge, K. A. (1994). A review and reformulation of social information-processing mechanisms in children's social adjustment. *Psychological Bulletin, 115,* 74–101. http://dx.doi.org/10.1037/0033-2909.115.1.74

Davidson, L., Stayner, D. A., Nickou, C., Styron, T. H., Rowe, M., & Chinman, M. L. (2001). "Simply to be let in": Inclusion as a basis for recovery. *Psychiatric Rehabilitation Journal, 24,* 375–388.

DeCarlo, J. J., & Mann, W. C. (1985). The effectiveness of verbal versus activity groups in improving self-perceptions of interpersonal communication skills. *American Journal of Occupational Therapy, 39,* 20–27. http://dx.doi.org/10.5014/ajot.39.1.20

Deci, E. L., & Ryan, R. M. (2000). The what and why of goal pursuits: Human needs and self-determination of behavior. *Psychological Inquiry, 11,* 227–268. http://dx.doi.org/10.1207/S15327965PLI1104_01

Devine, J., Cohen, J., & Elias, M. J. (2007). *Making your school safe: Strategies to protect children and protect children and promote learning.* New York: Columbia University.

Donohue, M. V. (1982). Designing activities to develop a women's identification group. *Occupational Therapy in Mental Health, 2,* 1–19. http://dx.doi.org/10.1300/J004v02n01_01

Duncombe, L. W., & Howe, M. C. (1995). Group treatment: Goals, tasks, and economic implications. *American Journal of Occupational Therapy, 49,* 199–205, discussion 206. http://dx.doi.org/10.5014/ajot.49.3.199

Elias, M. E., O'Brien, M. U., & Weissberg, R. P. (2006). Transformative leadership for social emotional learning. *Principal Leadership, 7,* 10–13.

Fiese, B. H. (2007). Routines and rituals: Opportunities for participation in family health. *OTJR: Occupation, Participation and Health, 27,* 41–49.

Fontana, D. (1990). *Social skills at work.* New York: Wiley-Blackwell.

Foot, H., Morgan, M., & Shute, R. (Eds.). (1990). *Children helping children.* London: Wiley.

Gbowee, L., & Mithers, C. (2011). *Mighty be our powers: How sisterhood, prayer, and sex changed a nation at war.* New York: Beast Books.

Greenberg, M. T., & Kusche, C. A. (1998). *Promoting alternative teaching strategies.* Boulder: University of Colorado, Institute of Behavioral Sciences.

Gutman, S. A., McCreedy, P., & Heisler, P. (2004). The psychosocial deficits of children with regulatory disorders: Identification and treatment. *Occupational Therapy in Mental Health, 20,* 1–32. http://dx.doi.org/10.1300/J004v20n02_01

Haglund, L., & Henriksson, C. (2003). Concepts in occupational therapy in relation to the ICF. *Occupational Therapy International, 10,* 253–268. http://dx.doi.org/10.1002/oti.189

Hayes, J. (2002). *Interpersonal skills at work.* New York: Routledge.

Hinojosa, J., Kramer, P., & Crist, P. (Eds.). (2010). *Evaluation: Obtaining and interpreting data* (3rd ed.). Bethesda, MD: AOTA Press.

Isaksson, G., Lexell, J., & Skar, L. (2007). Social support provides motivation and ability to participate in occupation. *OTJR: Occupation, Participation and Health, 27,* 23–30.

Jackson, L. L., & Arbesman, M. (2005). *Occupational therapy practice guidelines for children with behavioral and psychosocial needs.* Bethesda, MD: AOTA Press.

Jetten, J., Haslam, C., & Haslam, A. (Eds.). (2012). *The social cure: Identity, health and well being.* New York: Psychology Press.

Johnson, D. W., & Johnson, F. P. (2009). *Joining together: Group theory and group skills.* Boston: Allyn & Bacon.

Kam, C. M., Greenberg, M. T., & Kusche, C. A. (2004). Sustained effects of the PATHS curriculum on the social and psychological adjustment of children in special education. *Journal of Emotional and Behavioral Disorders, 12,* 66–78. http://dx.doi.org/10.1177/10634266040120020101

Kanas, N. (1966). *Group therapy for schizophrenic patients.* Washington, DC: American Psychiatric Press.

Kaplan, K. L. (1988). *Directive group therapy: Innovative mental health treatment.* Thorofare, NJ: Slack.

Kielhofner, G. (2006). *Research in occupational therapy: Methods of inquiry for enhancing practice.* Philadelphia: F. A. Davis.

Kim, J., Kim, S. Y., & Kaslak, M. A. (2005). Teachers' understanding and uses of developmentally appropriate practice for young children in Korea. *Journal of Research in Childhood Education, 20,* 49–56. http://dx.doi.org/10.1080/02568540509594550

Kramer, P., & Hinojosa, J. (2009). *Frames of reference for pediatric occupational therapy* (3rd ed.). New York: Lippincott Williams & Wilkins.

Lifton, W. M. (1966). *Working with groups: Group process and individual growth.* New York: Wiley.

Lisina, M. I. (1985). *Child–adults–peers: Patterns of communication.* Moscow: Progress.

Moos, R. H. (1994). *Group Environment Scale manual: Development, applications, research.* Palo Alto, CA: Consulting Psychologists Press.

Nelson, D. L., Melville, L. L., Wilkerson, J. D., Magness, R. A., Grech, J. L., & Rosenberg, J. A. (2002). Interrater reliability, concurrent validity, responsiveness, and predictive validity of the Melville–Nelson Self-Care Assessment. *American Journal of Occupational Therapy, 56,* 51–59. http://dx.doi.org/10.5014/ajot.56.1.51

Neufeld, P. S. (2004, August 9). Enabling participation through community and population approaches. *OT Practice,* pp. CE1–CE8.

O'Neil, H., & Perez, R. (Eds.). (2007). *Computer games and team and individual learning.* Los Angeles: Elsevier Science.

Ornish, D. (1999). *Love and survival.* New York: Harper Perennial.

Passi, L. E. (1998). *A guide to creative group programming in the psychiatric day hospital.* Binghamton, NY: Haworth Press.

Polit, D. F., & Hungler, B. P. (1995). *Nursing research: Principles and methods.* Philadelphia: Lippincott.

Posthuma, B. W. (2002). *Small groups in counseling and therapy: Process and leadership* (4th ed.). Needham Heights, MA: Allyn & Bacon.

Precin, P. (1999). *Living skills recovery workbook.* Boston: Butterworth Heinemann.

Putnam, R. (1993). The prosperous community: Social capital and public life. *American Prospect, 13,* 35–42.

Putnam, R. (1995). Bowling alone: America's declining social capital. *Journal of Democracy, 6,* 65–78. http://dx.doi.org/10.1353/jod.1995.0002

Putnam, R. (1996). The strange disappearance of civic America. *American Prospect, 24,* 1–15.

Putnam, R. (2000). *Bowling alone: The collapse and renewal of American community.* New York: Simon & Schuster.

Raphael-Greenfield, E., Shteyler, A., Silva, M. R., Canine, P. G., Soo, S., Rotonda, E. C., & Patrone, D. O. (2011). Hard-wired for groups: Students and clients in the classroom and clinic. *Mental Health Special Interest Quarterly, 34,* 1–4.

Remocker, A. J., & Sherwood, E. T. (1999). *Action speaks louder: A handbook of structured group techniques* (6th ed.). New York: Churchill Livingston.

Robinson, C. C., Anderson, G. T., Porter, C. L., Hart, C. H., & Wouden-Miller, M. (2003). Sequential patterns in the natural play of preschool children: Is parallel play a bridge to other play states. *Early Childhood Research Quarterly, 18,* 3–21. http://dx.doi.org/10.1016/S0885-2006(03)00003-6

Ross, M. (1997). *Integrative group therapy: Mobilizing coping abilities with the five stage group.* Bethesda, MD: American Occupational Therapy Association.

Sampson, E. E., & Marthas, M. (1990). *Group process for the health professions* (3rd ed.). New York: Delmar Cengage Learning.

Sanders, C., & Phye, G. (Eds.). (2004). *Bullying: Implications for the classroom.* New York: Academic Press.

Schultz, J., & Reilly, R. (2006). *It's all part of the job: Social skills for success at work.* Birmingham, AL: Attainment.

Schutz, P., Pekrum, R., & Phye, G. (2007). *Emotion in education.* New York: Academic Press.

Schwartzberg, S. L. (2002). *Interactive reasoning in the practice of occupational therapy.* Upper Saddle River, NJ: Prentice Hall.

Schwartzberg, S. L., Howe, M. C., & Barnes, M. A. (2008). *Groups: Applying the functional group model.* Philadelphia: F. A. Davis.

Schwartzberg, S. L., Howe, M., & McDermott, A. (1982). A comparison of three treatment group formats for facilitating social interaction. *Occupational Therapy in Mental Health, 2,* 1–16.

Simon, S. B., Howe, L. W., & Kirshenbaum, H. (1992). *Values clarification: A handbook of practical strategies for teachers and students* (rev. ed.) New York: Hart.

Sladyk, K., Jacobs, K., & MacCrae, N. (Eds.). (2010). *Occupational therapy essentials for clinical competence.* Thorofare, NJ: Slack.

Social Capital Foundation. (2008). *Mission statement.* Available at www.socialcapital-foundation.org/TSCF/TSCF%20mission_statement.html

Swarbrick, M. (2009). Peer-operated services: A resource for mental health system transformation. *Occupational Therapy in Mental Health, 25,* 343–351. http://dx.doi.org/10.1080/01642120903083945

Tsang, H. W.-H., & Pearson, V. (2001). Work-related social skills training for people with schizophrenia in Hong Kong. *Schizophrenia Bulletin, 27,* 139–148. http://dx.doi.org/10.1093/oxfordjournals.schbul.a006852

Ward, K., Mitchell, J., & Price, P. (2007). Occupation-based practice and its relationship to social and occupational participation in adults with spinal cord injury. *OTJR: Occupation, Participation and Health, 27,* 149–156.

World Health Organization. (2007). *International classification of functioning, disability and health: Children and youth version (ICF–CY).* Geneva: Author.

Yalom, I. D., & Leszcz, M. (2005). *The theory and practice of group psychotherapy* (5th ed.). New York: Basic Books.

Zins, J. E., Elias, M. J., & Maher, C. A. (Eds.). (2007). *Bullying victimization and peer harassment: A handbook of prevention and intervention.* Binghamton, NY: Haworth Press.

Zins, J. E. Weissberg, R. P., Wang, M. C., & Walberg, H. J. (Eds.). (2004). *Building academic success on social and emotional learning: What does the research say?* New York: Teachers College Press.